Look to

——— Dr. Spock's The School Years ———

for invaluable advice to parents on successfully raising a
child to young adulthood:

- Teaching values and responsibilities
- Sibling rivalry
- Education
- Discipline and punishme'
- Drug, alcohol, and vio'
- Peer pressure and r
- Activities and socia.

. . . and more!

BOOKS BY BENJAMIN SPOCK, M.D.

Dr. Spock's Baby and Child Care
Dr. Spock on Parenting
Dr. Spock's The First Two Years
Dr. Spock's The School Years

Published by POCKET BOOKS

Dr. Spock's

THE
SCHOOL
YEARS

The Emotional and
Social Development of Children

Benjamin Spock, M.D.
edited by Martin T. Stein, M.D.

POCKET BOOKS
New York   London   Toronto   Sydney   Singapore

An *Original* Publication of POCKET BOOKS

 POCKET BOOKS, a division of Simon & Schuster, Inc.
1230 Avenue of the Americas, New York, NY 10020

ISBN: 0-7434-1123-4

First Pocket Books trade paperback printing August 2001

10 9 8 7 6 5 4 3 2 1

POCKET and colophon are registered trademarks of
Simon & Schuster, Inc.

Front cover photo by VCG/FPG International

Printed in the U.S.A.

This book is comprised of a series of essays previously published individually in
Redbook (1985–1992) and *Parenting* (1992–1998).

For information regarding special discounts for bulk purchases, please
contact Simon & Schuster Special Sales at 1-800-456-6798 or
business@simonandschuster.com

This book is dedicated to

the mothers and fathers who taught Dr. Spock about the growth and emotional development of their children;

Dr. Benjamin Spock, who shared with me, during the last year of his remarkable life, the evolution of his ideas about the development of children;

Mary Morgan, Dr. Spock's widow, who steadfastly maintains his legacy for the children and parents of future generations;

my parents, Gertrude and Gerald Stein, who guided the lives of their children with a respect for their independence and an intuitive understanding of Dr. Spock's reminder to parents to "trust yourself . . . you know more than you think you do," and

my wife, Mary Caffery, and children, Joshua, Benjamin, and Sarah, who continue to teach me about the developmental journey of children and young adults.

Acknowledgments

There are many individuals who are important in the development of this book. I am indebted to the pediatricians who shaped my thinking about children, families, and the practice of pediatrics, including Drs. John Castiglione, Louis Fraad, William Nyhan, Samuel Spector, Stanford Friedman, John Kennell, and T. Berry Brazelton. I especially want to thank my colleague Dr. Suzanne Dixon, with whom I collaborated during a twenty-year period at the University of California San Diego.

There are many other colleagues in the emerging specialty of Developmental and Behavioral Pediatrics who continue to work with me and teach me about ways to assist pediatricians to become more effective in counseling parents and in the early recognition and treatment of children with developmental and behavioral conditions. They include Drs. Michael Reiff, Heidi Feldman, Ellen Perrin, Paul Dworkin, William Coleman, Lane Tanner, Jim Perrin, Mark Wolraich, Esther

Wender, William Carey, Ronald Barr, Randi Hagerman, Barbara Howard, Robert Needlman, and David Snyder. My colleagues in San Diego—Philip Nader, Laurel Leslie, Barbara Loundsbury, Dorothy Johnson, Eyla Boies, and Howard Taras—continue to support this work.

I also wish to express sincere appreciation to Robert Lescher, Dr. Spock's literary agent for many years. He steadfastly encouraged and guided the publication of this book. Dr. Spock wrote the original articles included in the book for two magazines. Bruce Raskin encouraged and guided the publication as Dr. Spock's editor at *Parenting* magazine, and Sylvia Koner was his editor at *Redbook*. I am also grateful to Tracy Bernstein, a superb editor at Pocket Books.

Dr Benjamin Spock's legacy is sustained today at drspock.com, a company that disseminates his writings and contemporary information for parents. The leadership of that group worked with me and actively encouraged the development of this book. I appreciate the support from Douglas Lee, John Buckley, David Markus, George Strait, and Drs. Laura Janna, Robert Needlman, and Lynn Cates.

Contents

Introduction   **xiii**

1. **Teaching Values to Children**   **1**

    Teaching Children to Give and Share   1

    Duties and Responsibilities   9

    Do Kids Have Too Much?   13

    Rising Stresses and Weakening Spirituality   19

    Children and Religion   39

    Causes for Children   42

    Violence in the News, Movies, and on Television   47

2. **Families**   **60**

    The Changing Family   60

    Early or Late Childbearing   66

    The Second Child   72

    Loving One Child Less   78

    Preparing Children for a Good Marriage   81

Can One Parent Be as Good as Two?   88

The Pains of a Stepparent   98

Are Grandparents Important?   105

The Interfering Grandmother   111

Vacation Without the Children   118

Trying to Keep the Holidays Relaxed   125

3. **Contemporary Culture**   **130**

Changes in the Care of Children and
Old People   130

Can You Raise Children to Make Their Own
Decisions?   134

Parental Guilt from Working
Outside the Home   141

Children Speak Out About Scheduling   146

Calling Parents by First Names   152

Teenage Idols, Punk Style, and the
Early Stages of Sexual Development   157

How Open Can You Be About Sex?   164

4. **Discipline: Teaching Children Expectations
for Behavior**   **174**

Hesitancy in Parents   174

Consistency in Discipline   184

The Father's Role in Discipline   186

Lying   190

5. **The Social Development of Children**   **197**

Play: The "Work" of Early Childhood   197

Sibling Rivalry   205

How to Help a Child Who Isn't Popular 210

Peer Pressure in Adolescence 216

Compare and Despair 226

The Neighbors' Kids 231

6. **Education** **239**

What Is Education? 239

Incidental Learning 245

Competitiveness 250

How Can You Judge Your Child's Teacher? 258

Lessons, Lessons 264

Index **269**

Introduction

For nearly seventy years, from the 1930s to the end of the twentieth century, Dr. Benjamin Spock was *the* pediatrician to whom parents turned for guidance about a wide variety of child rearing issues. The popularity of his first book, *Baby and Child Care*, brought national and international recognition to Dr. Spock for his sound, practical advice and gentle voice. It became the most widely read book on child care ever written.

Today, decades later, it is still the most respected parenting book in the world; and Dr. Spock's other books are equally celebrated. Although he is gone, millions of parents continue to "consult" him by virtue of his writings. Why such popularity and success? I think there are three major reasons.

First, his range of subjects was comprehensive, incorporating parents' concerns about physical health (for example, nutrition, safety, immunizations, early signs of illness, and home remedies) and psychological health (knowledge about normal development, parent and sibling relationships, the different experiences of mothers and fathers, the effect of work outside the home on family life, and many others).

Second, a hallmark of his writing is that Dr. Spock "spoke" to parents. Mothers and fathers often wrote to him with some variation of "When I read your book, it is as if you are sitting at my kitchen table talking and listening to me." His focus was always on the parent; he wrote with the assumption that parents are capable, wise, and open to understanding the development and needs of their children. "Trust yourself" was a theme that guided all of his advice to parents.

The third reason, I believe, for the preeminent place Dr. Spock continues to hold among parents is his respect for change and diversity. He recognized that the way we raise children reflects a culture's values and that some of our values and perspectives on children and family change over time. Characteristically, he did not tell us "the right way to do it." He recognized the inherent value of diversity in families and communities. In every position he took, he respected that diversity.

This book derives from a series of articles published in two magazines, *Redbook* (1985–1992) and *Parenting* (1992–1998). The articles have been edited, catalogued, and published in two volumes.

Dr. Spock's The School Years explores current trends in our society that have an impact on raising children. It is published with a companion volume, *Dr. Spock's The First*

Two Years, the table of contents for which can be found at the end of the book.

Dr. Spock begins with a discussion of the values he believed are most important to instill, including teaching children to give and share and the value of duties and responsibilities at an early age. He explores our current emphasis on material things by asking the question "Do kids have too much?" and asserts the importance of spirituality in the emerging value system of children. Dr. Spock's definition of spirituality is broad: "By spiritual values I mean generosity, kindness, cooperation, honesty, the creation and appreciation of beauty, idealism, love. . . . I am writing primarily about aspects of spirituality that don't depend on religious beliefs, but rather a spirituality that applies to people's relationships with each other and with themselves, whether or not they are religious."

The next section begins with a discussion of the changing family. Dr. Spock deeply respected all those who care for children, not just the traditional nuclear family with two parents. The single parent, divorced parents, parents who raise children in stepfamilies, and stepparents are all appreciated for what they bring to child-rearing, as are the contributions of grandparents. In "Preparing children for a good marriage," Dr. Spock points out that children learn about respect, love, and how to act in a decent way by watching their parents.

The section on contemporary culture explores many current concerns of parents, including the enormous challenges of working parents, the risk of overscheduling a child's activities, the influence of television, and the uncertainties of adolescent sexuality. Throughout his writings, and particularly in this section, he addresses the necessity of raising children who can make their own decisions.

The next two sections, on discipline and social development, are applicable for parents with both young and older children. Discipline is understood as an opportunity to teach children expectations for behavior, beginning in infancy and continuing through adolescence. Dr. Spock believed that hesitancy in parenting was the major barrier to effective discipline. He helps parents understand the many factors that seem to encourage hesitancy and makes suggestions for improvement. Other topics include lying, the importance of play, popularity, peer pressure and sibling rivalry.

Another central concern that runs throughout Dr. Spock's writings is the importance of education, which in his definition extended beyond the classroom to include activities with family members and peers, in the home and in the community. In the final section of the book, he highlights the value of a warm, mutually respectful relationship between teacher and student, and the significance of human relations as a core component of all education. He concludes with some specific recommendations of how public education could be improved to better meet the needs of children.

During the year prior to his recent death, Dr. Spock and I met several times each week. With his wife, Mary

Morgan, he had moved from the colder climate of his beloved Maine to southern California, a more gentle climate at a time of declining health. Sitting in his patio surrounded by many plants, colorful flowers, a large aquarium and a canyon view covered with green chaparral, we talked about children. Together, we reviewed the seventh edition of *Baby and Child Care*. I was amazed at his enthusiasm. At ninety-four years of age, with a weakening physical body, he found the intellectual and emotional strength to engage and be engaged in a dialogue about ideas that remained important to him. New approaches to encourage and sustain breast feeding, eliminating the traditional use of powder for diaper rashes, aspects of his new recommendation for a vegetarian diet, and reviewing newer approaches to bed-wetting are a few examples of subjects we discussed. Dr. Spock's thoughtful responses were consistently laced with his clinical experiences and the ideas and suggestions he gleaned from the many parents who wrote to him.

When I read the essays collected in this book I hear that voice. It is a voice that comes from an informed and thoughtful mind, a voice that speaks directly to parents—with confidence in your wish to be a good parent. He trusted and respected your intelligence and good intentions. It is my hope that this book captures the knowledge and wisdom of a pediatrician who dedicated his life to the emotional and physical health of children.

1

Teaching Values to Children

Teaching Children to Give and Share

Real generosity can't be taught in the way the multiplication tables can be taught, by telling and by drilling. For generosity is much more fundamental than just the polite sharing of playthings with friends or giving presents to relatives on their birthdays. Real generosity springs from love, the deepest, strongest, and most durable of the emotions. If children aren't loving, efforts to teach them to share and give won't accomplish much.

But even children who have plenty of love in their hearts will need some help in expressing it as generosity. And they'll be more ready to learn at certain stages of childhood, and under certain conditions, which parents should know about.

Children are born equipped to learn to love, at the

appropriate stages, in response to their parents' love. When parents have no love to give, their children never become loving. Love is expressed by parents—and appreciated by children—in various ways at different ages. Toward very young infants, parents show it by being ever ready to comfort them when they are miserable—for example, with hunger or cold or fatigue or the belly ache. Young babies learn to trust and appreciate this faithfulness. We know this by comparing the development of babies who have been raised by responsive and loving parents with babies raised by unreliable, unfeeling parents.

As babies grow, their parents shower them with smiles, hugs, exaggerated compliments, and baby talk. You can see the effect in the delight with which these babies respond.

In the second and third years, children feel the urge to independence: they insist on their right to make certain decisions and to say *No.* Yet at the same time they become much more aware of their need for dependence on their parents. They fear separation from them. They are leery of strangers. Loving parents tactfully show their awareness of both these opposite needs: They never let them feel abandoned; they let them think they are winning some of the arguments, and avoid others altogether.

Between the ages of three and six children seem to feel that they've achieved enough independence for the time being; they become less argumentative, more outgoing, more cooperative, more companionable.

Their most powerful drive now is to pattern themselves after their parents whom they admire extravagantly. They want to speak like them, dress like them, play at the same occupations as far as they can, pretend to be married and have babies of their own, just like their parents. Children's outgoingness and affectionateness at this age make them ready to learn sharing and giving—and to enjoy them.

After the age of six years, children feel a renewed urge toward independence. They no longer want slavishly to identify with parents. They turn to children of their own age and sex to identify with, to speak like them, dress like them, have the same playthings, hobbies, and ideals. They are beginning a crucial shift—from being a child of the family to being a person of the outer world.

Now let's look more closely at the readiness for generosity at different ages. Even before a year of age, a baby chewing on a crust of bread will offer the soggy end to his mother, with a smile that's both loving and proud. He's proud to be copying such a grown-up act, I think. His mother encourages his generosity by smacking her lips over this morsel. At a little over one year, a baby just able to walk will keep his distance from his mother's visitor while he scrutinizes her carefully for a quarter or half an hour, as if to discover whether she is safe to approach. He is now both scared and eager to make friends. He decides he likes her, walks slowly up to her, and offers her one of his precious toys, perhaps even his favorite comforter. She reaches out and he allows her to take hold of it. But he doesn't let go. I'd say that he has the impulse to be generous but that giving up a personal possession is still way beyond him. This may seem perplexing to an adult, who thinks of offering and letting go as two stages of the same process.

By two years of age, children are watching their parents and imitating any action they can manage, particularly anything that seems helpful such as fetching a diaper for the new baby or putting the knives, forks, and spoons on the table. I knew a two-year-old who even offered his precious pacifier to the new baby, an act of extreme generosity! But such feelings may be ended abruptly when the baby grows old enough to begin grabbing the older child's possessions.

This spontaneous helpfulness toward the parents or a dependent baby is quite different from sharing toys with other children of the same age or playing cooperatively with them. In fact, this is still the age period when a child indignantly cries out *Mine* when another child tries to use his possession and goes after him to fiercely yank it away. Or he may bat the other child with the toy or bite him.

Two-year-olds enjoy watching other children play and imitating them. This is sometimes called parallel play; but it shouldn't be confused with cooperative play or sharing.

Now let's get on to how you can help children to be givers. It goes without saying that they should feel well loved—from birth to adulthood. Parental love is more than hugs and baby talk, of course. It's meeting children's legitimate needs for physical affection, for appreciation of their achievements, for comforting when they are hurt in body or spirit. It's sensing that they'll probably be made jealous by the arrival of a brother or sister and talking with them sympathetically about their mixed feelings.

Parental love has to include sensible control as children grow old enough to get into trouble or to hurt other people's possessions. But control doesn't have to include punishment or disagreeableness, only firmness and reasonable consistency.

The most useful advice I can offer about fostering generosity is to take full advantage of the impulse in children at different ages to be helpful and giving. Lay your hand on the toy half offered by the one-year-old; smile and say thank you three times, but don't try to get the toy away from him—that would bring out his possessiveness.

Welcome the helpfulness of the two-year-old who wants to put the eating utensils on the table. Don't say to him or to yourself that you can do it faster yourself. That's not the point. The time to let children help you—or help themselves—is when it seems exciting to them (provided, of course, that it's not dangerous). If you put them off until they are more skilled, the impulse will have passed and you'll have to persuade them or make them do what's no longer appealing. Express appreciation for a job well done. Keep holding out the hope that someday they'll be able to take on a more difficult job, like putting the plates on the table.

Don't try to persuade two-year-olds to share their playthings with others. They are too possessive to accept the idea. They may already be suspicious that other children are trying to get their playthings. When their parents urge them to share, they feel that everyone is out to rob them. This may make them more possessive than ever.

As children get into the three-to-five year-old stage, they become more outgoing. They enjoy each other's company. They are more ready for cooperative play, in which they build block structures together or play "house" or doctor and patient, or pretend to be driver and passengers in a bus, or take turns pulling the wagon and riding in it. To help them make this transition from selfish to generous, parents can demonstrate the fun of cooperative play, by entering in, enthusiastically. Such suggestions are much more likely to fall on receptive soil at three years than at two. This is the time to encourage wider, regular participation in housework and yard work by showing appreciation and making suggestions in a cordial spirit.

Make the times, when you and the child are working together, social occasions when you chat and gossip enjoyably, as you would do with an adult friend.

If a child forgets to be helpful one day, resist the impulse to scold. Remind her how much she helps you and how much you need her help today. If this fails, be a bit more insistent, without getting cross. Remember that in day-care centers they expect and get housekeeping help from the children, week after week, all year long!

After the age of six years, children turn away from their fascination with playing "house"—which is playing family—and with playing at marriage and caring for babies. Their interests are now science, nature, school work, hobbies. They no longer want to identify with their parents. Instead they identify with their peers—in their language, clothes, table manners, and possessions. They are concerned with how to be accepted in the school and in the community.

In their devotion to their pals they are likely to form clubs or gangs, one of the main functions of which is to exclude those who seem different. So there is a strong trend toward intolerance, which can be quite cruel. On the other hand, children are eager to find out how things are done in the outside world. If they have parents and teachers whom they respect because they are wise but kind, they can be easily led into understanding and feeling friendly toward people from other backgrounds and other parts of the world. I was impressed with how my two children, who had loving, socially conscious teachers, became increasingly tolerant and appreciative of other kinds of people as they progressed though the grades. This spirit is still very prominent in their adult years. I consider tolerance to be a vital aspect of generosity, which can certainly be taught, by both teachers and parents, and which will help their children to get along throughout their social and occupational lives.

After six and through the teen years, children can be encouraged to think generously of those outside their own circle. They can repair, with a parent's help, toys they have outgrown that may be collected and distributed to disadvantaged children by some local organization. They can donate a nominal part of their allowance or earnings at Sunday school or to another charity. As adolescents they can volunteer for community service such as offering books or singing in groups to adult hospital patients, playing with or reading to children in hospitals and other institutions, or tutoring younger pupils in school.

I want to make a special plea for generosity at Christmas, Chanukah, and birthdays. These are occasions when many children are encouraged to nearly wallow in greediness. They think and talk only about what they want. I think also that many of them get too many gifts. Parents have the opportunity to shift the emphasis somewhat. Encourage your children to make their own holiday greeting cards, and simple presents for their parents and grandparents. Let them think about, choose and pay for the presents for their friends at the birthday party and for friends and young relatives for Christmas and for Chanukah.

Children are no different than adults in getting joy from giving. I can still remember vividly my satisfaction in third grade making a set of small blotters tied together with a ribbon, the top one embellished with a tiny calendar and a crayon drawing of a house in the snow. (When I was growing up, all the adults had to have blotters because the ink in pens dried slowly.) After I took it home, I hid it as carefully as if it was a diamond ring. On Christmas morning I could hardly wait for my parents to open it.

It's not only more blessed to give, it's more exciting. This is particularly true if the parents have emphasized this point of view and have demonstrated their joy in giving.

Duties and Responsibilities

At age two years, a child can begin helping to dress himself. Children are eager to do the grown-up thing. They will stay interested and stay at the job longer if the parent works with them.

I think the main thing you want to think about is the "spirit" with which you present duties and responsibilities. Young children are wild to be grown up. They follow older siblings around eager to imitate them. They play "house" all day where they take on the responsibility of caring for a doll. They are very eager to learn the responsibilities of adult life.

This eagerness and enthusiasm is the key ingredient as you begin to teach your child these duties. If you stay with this spirit, which the child has naturally, and show the same enthusiasm for the job and work along with the child, then it's a joy rather than a chore. If you leave it for the child to do alone, or you feel angry and demand that the child do these duties, then the spirit of excitement and enjoyment is crushed. And even though you may get the chore done quicker through threats, you have lost the real job, which is to have a cooperative and loving spirit both from the child and from the parent.

You can decide what chore you would like your child to learn, then be sure that she is capable of doing the chore. Let's say it's picking up her toys. If she's an eager three-year-old and sees that putting the toys away is part of "play," then she'll eagerly follow your lead. You can show her how to put the doll to bed in her crib each time, then she'll soon catch on that that's where the doll goes when she is finished playing. These habits can easily be formed without nagging. Of course, you can do the job much faster by yourself, but that misses the point. Fast isn't the goal here. It takes talking to the child and showing her how to put away her toys. You might say, "This is where your teddy likes to sleep when you are through playing with him." You must be patient with a child at this age, and realize they need to be reminded, but not scolded or nagged. And always working along with the child gives them an excellent role model. If you love what you do, your child will soon learn to love doing her job also.

When your child is a little older, you can begin teaching her simple food preparation. I know some children who were "cooking" and stirring food before they could walk. Your experience in the kitchen with your children can be very fulfilling, rewarding and fun. Be very careful with sharp knives with young children. But you'll find that young children love to pull up a chair to the sink and wash carrots. At six or seven years, they can fill a pot with water and prepare to steam or blanch the carrots. You can teach them to prepare peanut-butter sandwiches which they love.

Many children love to help plan a meal, shop for it, do the preparations, and serve it, following it through to completion. They may be forgetful at times, and I'm sure your kitchen will be messier, but the goal here is to help the child assume, in a joyful way, the preparation of food. This is a skill which your son or daughter will enjoy and use the rest of their life. So starting young can be a wonderful habit which you can both share. If you enjoy cooking and being in the kitchen, then your child will pick this up right away. If you hate to cook, then you should not even try to get your child to cook. Try instead some project that you can both feel some eagerness for.

If your two-year-old is eager to help out with the cooking, then she can stir the corn bread as you add the ingredients. And your older child can gradually cook the oatmeal, but only if you can be sure that she understands how to keep from burning herself. After she cooks it, she may want to serve it to herself and other family members, for further gratification.

The more you participate, in a cheerful and exciting manner, with your child in learning to do chores, the more success you will have. And you will find this a very rewarding experience as you learn patience, tolerate less tidiness, and accept the level of skill of your child. This can also be a very rewarding learning experience for the parents, as they learn from their child how to be patient and accepting.

Parents can best teach a child responsibility by being responsible themselves. Children love to model themselves after adults, and they will more likely show eagerness and readiness when the parents have responsibilities they take on with pride and joy.

When a child sees her father or mother raking the leaves, washing the car, or taking care of the lawn, then the child will want to put on her boots and get a brush and scrub the tires of the car, and rinse the car with the hose. She may spray herself as well, but she will enjoy the close companionship of her father or mother while doing a grown-up job.

Many children decide their careers early in life, and I'm sure that I decided to become a pediatrician because I was the oldest of six children, and I identified with my mother. I helped take care of my younger brother, Bob. And I changed diapers and gave bottles to my younger siblings. I'm sure that taking on the responsibilities of caring for my younger siblings gave me the foundation for going into pediatrics. When my mother would let me take care of one of the babies, I felt more grown up and identified with the adults, and acted like one too.

Parents sometimes find it hard to step back and let go and leave the doing of the job to the child, because the parent can do it faster and better. Your child's inexperience may try your patience, but you can give your child a sense of pride by showing that you have faith that she can do a good job.

DUTIES AND RESPONSIBILITIES—
SUGGESTIONS AT EACH AGE

Two-Year-Olds
- Set table—silverware
- Put napkins on table
- Help dress themselves

Three-Year-Olds
- Carry packages
- Pick up playthings (with help)
- Set table with silverware and dishes

Four-Year-Olds
- Empty waste baskets
- Learn to button
- Pick up toys

Five-Year-Olds
- Rake the lawn, along with parent (it's always good to work with parents)
- Tie shoelaces

Six-Year-Olds
- Help parent wash the car
- Feed the cat or dog

Seven-Year-Olds
- Make bed daily
- Take out the garbage
- Sweep or vacuum room weekly

Eight-Year-Olds
- Cook or prepare simple meals

Do Kids Have Too Much?

Many American children have a lot more possessions than children in other parts of the world. In infancy, a crib is usually full of stuffed animals. This pattern is followed throughout childhood with dolls, push-pull toys, a wagon, tricycle, toy cars, doll outfits, robots, guns, phonograph, table games, space ships, bicycle, athletic equipment, radio, perhaps a real car as a gift on the sixteenth birthday or earned with after-school jobs.

On speaking tours I usually stay with a family and am assigned to the child's room. In it there are so many playthings on bureau tops, shelves, and chairs that there is no room for my small toilet kit. And the closet is so tightly packed with clothes that there is no space or hanger for my jacket. (I'm not complaining, only making a point.) Parents in most other parts of the world would be flabbergasted or horrified by such indulgence.

Partly it's that the waves of people who've immigrated to the United States ever since 1620 uprooted themselves from the old country because they wanted their children to have all the advantages they themselves couldn't have—not just playthings but education, good jobs, religious freedom, and dignity.

I'm not thinking of playthings alone. Children can be indulged with too many clothes, too many privileges, too many parental sacrifices of any kind. It's not just the quantity or the expense of the things or the privileges. More important is the relationship of the cost to the parents' means. It's how much of a sacrifice they are making or being asked by the child to make, and most important of all, whether the child appreciates the sacrifice and shows a willingness to make some sacrifice, too.

For example, when a six-year-old asks for a bicycle, I think it's wise for the parents not to immediately go out and buy it. They can mention its expense and then discuss its appropriateness as a birthday, or Christmas, or Chanukah present. If these occasions are many months away, they can suggest that, by saving his allowance or performing a regular job, he can contribute his share to this major purchase. I feel that the delay in gratification and the sharing of the expense are both sensible in the case of something costly. It helps the child to understand that money doesn't grow on trees. It tests out whether his desire is a deep one or just a passing fancy. And it certainly makes him appreciate something that he has helped to pay for.

I think there is no doubt about it that, in general, children who have loads of possessions don't appreciate them as much as those who have only a moderate number. They come too easily, before the desire has had much chance to build up. More importantly, with fewer playthings, children are challenged to be creative, to think of new ways to vary their play—for example, to cast a doll in new roles, new situations, and to make the doll work through common difficulties in children's own lives, such as a fear of inoculations or resentment over punishments. In other words, the children have invested a lot more meaning in the plaything. I'm contrasting in my mind the American child almost swamped with toys and a child I saw in a documentary film about an undeveloped, poor country, playing endlessly with a doll she had fashioned out of a stick. It was all she had and she was making the most of it.

Another contrast, at the opposite extreme, is a situation occasionally seen in a child guidance clinic. The parents don't really love their child much, but in their guilt they heap presents on her instead, to try to make up for their lack of love. The gifts are not appreciated or played with. She may ignore them or even abuse them as she senses that they are substitutes for the love that she really wants.

Lack of parental love is rare. But it is fairly common for parents to overindulge their child because they feel guilty about something else. For example, they weren't ready for this pregnancy and hoped that it would terminate spontaneously. Or a son reminds the mother of the brother, whom she often treated meanly in childhood, because he seemed to her to be her parents' favorite. Or the parents, both of whom have full-time jobs, worry that they may be depriving their child.

Other parents overindulge because they want their children to have not only everything that the parents had but everything that they yearned for and didn't have. Others still are afraid to say no for fear they may be thought stingy by the neighbors or relatives or, occasionally, for fear their children will accuse them of lacking love.

Children are extremely sensitive to even slight guiltiness on their parents' part (as a matter of fact, they are sensitive to most parental moods) and they can't resist the temptation to take advantage of it. So they ask or beg or whine or bargain or demand. If they find that some such approach works, they'll keep at it until they have whatever they desire at the moment or until the parents resist firmly and confidently.

What has the undesirable effect on children is not so much the excess amount of possessions and privileges they may have but the feeling they may get that they can bully or badger or nag their parents into giving them more than the parents feel like giving or more than the parents feel is reasonable. It undermines their respect for their parents and for themselves.

There are various characteristics that such children may develop. They may, to some degree, become argumentative, greedy, self-centered, ungrateful, insensitive to the needs and feelings of others.

When children find that they can always pressure a parent into giving them more than is reasonable or fair, it makes them chronically guilty and cranky. They sense it's not right, that they should show more respect, and that they need limits (as we all do). The paradoxical result is that they push further, hoping subconsciously that they will eventually find some kind of parental limits. When they are locked into a too-demanding relationship with the parents, they may fail to develop fully various aspects of their own independence such as initiative, industriousness, creativity, and a sense of responsibility.

As they grow up, these children may not develop the capacity to please and play cooperatively with other children. When they are increasingly spending time with other children in the school years and sense that their popularity is impaired, they may either be able to wise-up about their selfishness and make an adjustment, at least with other children their own age, or they may go on antagonizing them.

It is hard on parents, too, when they can't stand up to their children's unreasonable demands. They vacillate between saying no and giving in. Neither position satisfies them for long. After they've said no, they feel a wave of remorse for having been so ungenerous. If they've given in, they are apt to feel regret and resentment over having been a pushover, for lacking the courage of their convictions.

This kind of vacillation impairs not only the parents' ability to sense limits. It destabilizes or sours the whole relationship to at least a slight degree, robbing it of some of the happiness, mutual respect, confidence in each other, and comfort that families are entitled to.

The real purpose of this discussion has not been to tell parents how much or how little to buy for their children, for circumstances are different in every family. It has been to help those parents who sense that they overindulge their children to see that this is not healthy for anyone and doesn't bring happiness to anyone.

Parents who are fortunate enough to have no problem with guilt or a submissive parenting style don't have to act severe or cross. They simply know their own minds. When their child asks for some possession or privilege that the parents feel does not justify immediate granting, they explain cheerfully that it's too expensive, except perhaps for a birthday or holiday gift, or unless the child is willing to contribute from allowance or jobs.

It's the cheerfulness and the lack of hesitation that impresses the child that the parent means it. A crabby response signals that the parent is already in inner conflict. I believe that most children abide by what their parents sincerely, clearly believe is right. What sets them to arguing and pestering is when they detect uncertainty and vacillation.

But, you may answer, I often am uncertain. That doesn't mean you can't change. First you try to figure out what makes you act submissive or guilty. Then, whether or not you've found the explanation, you have to practice prompt, friendly firmness.

When you turn over a new leaf, you can't expect to be consistently different right away. You have to be satisfied with gradual improvement, with ups and downs. And even after you are handling things much better, you can't expect the children to respond immediately. For a while, they'll keep on trying the old pressures that used to work so well. But they'll come around if you stick to your guns.

Rising Stresses and Weakening Spirituality

There are greater tensions bearing down on American parents and children than ever before, in my experience. They come from the state of our society as a whole—the stresses and the loss of spiritual values. By

spiritual values I mean generosity, kindliness, cooperation, honesty, the creation and appreciation of beauty,
idealism, love.

I want to make it clear at the start that I am writing
primarily about aspects of spirituality that don't depend
on religious beliefs, but rather a spirituality that applies
to people's relationships with each other and with themselves, whether or not they are religious. It includes dedication to family; working for a better country and better world; generosity and loyalty and love for relatives,
friends and fellow workers; honesty and fair dealing;
and holding to principles that others can count on.

When I think about the stresses on children and families today and their effect on spiritual values, I recall my
own childhood in a middle-class neighborhood in New
Haven, Connecticut. There was no word or thought of
murder, rape, wife or child abuse, teenage pregnancy, or
drugs. There must have been cases but not enough to be
dramatized in the newspapers. Discipline was strict. Life
was calm, almost humdrum. My father, a railroad lawyer,
came home for lunch everyday in the trolley car. He was
never threatened with unemployment; it was assumed
that professional men such as he, who worked hard and
saved, would surely have enough for retirement. My
mother gave birth to her six children at home and took
total care of us, as all middle-class parents did. She visited
her mother for tea everyday, pushing her latest in a baby
carriage, and we children were expected to play outdoors
until each was invited in by Nanny, for one cookie.

Of course, there was no radio or television. After

school we played in the backyard or, on rainy days, read any of the hundreds of classics provided by my mother—Mark Twain, Stevenson, Dickens, Thackeray, Kingsley, *The Book of Knowledge.*

The individual stresses today are well enough known; but I want to list them together, to bring out the multiplicity of the problems we face.

I wouldn't call attention to all these difficulties though unless I believed they could be overcome—not by going backward in time but by raising our children with a different emphasis and by also using political pressure to get government and industry to meet the needs that we can't satisfy as individuals. I know both can be done, from observing children raised in different ways, and from my political experiences in opposing the Vietnam war.

In the first place most of us no longer have the security and the comfort that used to come from living close to other members of our extended families—grandparents, aunts, uncles, cousins—and in small close-knit communities where most people knew each other and were ready to help each other in crises. It's said that in parts of Los Angeles people move on the average of once every eighteen months. How can anyone put down roots or draw comfort from the community when they have to keep moving at this rate?

Not as many people now feel that they have a personal, intimate relationship with a God who watches over them and guides them. And science has narrowed the authority of religion. What are the major events in the past few years that create stress on children and families and is especially challenging in the face of a weakening spirituality?

PARENTS WORKING OUTSIDE OF THE HOME

Nowadays half the mothers and fathers of preschool children feel obliged—most for financial reasons—to work outside the home. Women have as much right as men to a career. But we haven't solved the problem of who is going to take care of the young children. It's fine if there's a willing grandmother or aunt, or if the parents can dovetail their work schedules; but few have these advantages. In my childhood, only the wealthy had live-in "children's nurses." Working mothers had to use "day nurseries," which provided only inadequate custodial care.

We now know that high-quality day care—meaning few children per teacher who is well trained in the care and education of young children—substitutes reasonably well for good parental care, but we don't have nearly enough of such care. And it's too expensive for a majority of parents. Meanwhile thousands of children, hundreds of thousands really, are being emotionally deprived by mediocre care at a crucial stage of development. This leaves parents feeling chronically guilty and dissatisfied because they know that the care is not as good as they'd like.

It's shameful that in the richest country the world has ever known we are shortchanging our children.

Our government says that it can't afford to subsidize day care. Nonsense! It is still spending trillions for unnecessary arms. All European countries and Canada do better than ours. Industry is just beginning to provide day care; it is worth their while, just from the point of view of employee loyalty and productivity.

DIVORCE AND CHILDREN

I'm not against divorce. I was divorced myself. But we have to realize what a strain it creates on every member of the family. All children of divorced families develop symptoms such as fears, bad dreams, aggressiveness, depression, and poor school work that may last for at least two years. It's hard on parents, particularly the custodial parents. It is of some help to parents to know ahead of time that they and their children are going to experience some of these symptoms. Then they can decide whether and how best to divorce, or try harder to make the marriage work.

There are probably many explanations including the fact that increasing frequency of divorce makes for increasing social acceptance of it. In speaking to a singles club, where most members were divorced, I happened to ask how many wished they had tried longer and harder to make a go of their marriages, and about half of them raised a hand. This suggests that divorce is often decided on in anger, before all remedies have been explored, perhaps with the help of a counselor. I think that another factor may be that many of us today are preoccupied with what we need and want as individuals, rather than being geared primarily to think of what our obligations to children and society are.

Two people who once would do and say anything to please the other now will do or say anything to irritate or anger the other as long as they can justify it by what the other has done. It's within the power of both to please or displease, to wreck or heal the marriage.

After divorce, the majority remarry and then there are often the painful problems of the step-relationships. Years ago I wrote an article about how to be a stepparent which I thought had a lot of wisdom in it. But when I became a stepparent I found that I didn't know how to follow the advice I had written. In my distress at the way I was rejected ("You're not my parent and I don't have to do what you say."), I did all the wrong things, such as scolding and disciplining, which only stimulate defiance.

WORK WITHOUT SATISFACTION

Another major problem we have, though we don't really think of it much, is that work for a majority of people is not satisfying except for the wages. Way back in simpler times, people made things like pots and jars and garments and quilts. They made them as beautiful as they could, whether they were going to use them or sell them. There is tremendous satisfaction to creating something whole and beautiful. I think of the time I constructed an eight-foot sailboat; it took me months and months, shaping the frame and the plywood, boring 360 little screw holes and inserting 360 little brass screws. But I didn't think it was boring work because all the time I had the vision of finishing a boat I could sail in. Finally I put on one coat of paint which covered the grime, and suddenly it turned clean and sleek-looking and I was filled with pride. It never leaked a drop. That's the kind of satisfaction our species was designed to get from work. But many of us have to turn to hobbies to get it.

At assembly lines in the factory, or in the office, workers sit hour after hour, month after month, repeating motions that have little meaning in themselves, whether it's assembling carburetors or filling out forms. It is simply a more efficient and profitable way to do things. But increasingly in recent years factory workers, in Europe as well as in America, have been complaining that this is a boring and a stressful way to make a living. As in so many aspects of our society—sports, art collecting, publishing—the amount of money to be made has taken over as the highest priority, displacing pleasure or the contribution that work brings to the society.

TOO MUCH COMPETITION

We have become an excessively competitive society and I blame this most of all for our tensions. I think the message that many parents give to their children is "Get ahead, kid, that's what you are in the world for." A distressing example is the effort to make super-kids. It was discovered, for instance, that if you could hold a child captive, and try hard enough, you could teach her to read at the age of two! The experimenter says he doesn't put any pressure on the child. But the child whom I saw in the film looked like a scared rabbit looking for a way to escape. All this effort and pressure without anybody ever having shown that if you learn to read at the age of two years, it's going to make you read any better at eight years than if you learned at six-years-old, the conventional age for learning to read! My own hunch is that you disturb the child by putting that amount of pressure on her, and you may make her dislike all schooling. In my school days teaching was cut and dried, which was not ideal, but it was better than intense pressure.

Most important in my opinion is to bring up our children with much less emphasis on getting ahead or on acquiring things. Parents can set the example by not overemphasizing their jobs at the expense of their families. I once had discussions with classes of eleven- and twelve-year-olds, most of whose parents were professionals or executives. They were proud of their parents' important jobs but were bitter about the small amount of time they had with them on workday nights or on weekends. They felt particularly deprived when parents explained that they were too busy to attend athletic events, music and dance recitals, and school plays in which their children participated.

Fathers and mothers with the best of intentions often help to form little leagues to teach sports and sportsmanship to young children. But I worry that in many cases this overemphasizes competitiveness, the striving for perfection, and the importance of winning at too young an age. I've seen a father, embarrassed by his son's mistake or blunder in a little league game, land on him much too scornfully. And I've heard of parents piling out of the grandstand to threaten the umpire over a decision. Parents used to send children to camp to study nature and have fun at sports. Now they often send them to specialize in computer science, algebra, or tennis camps.

All these pressures on children are only a reflection of the intense pressures that our society puts on ambitious parents, to gain affluence, prestige, and position. I've talked with fathers whose adolescent child has gotten into trouble who confessed that they had been so preoccupied with getting ahead at their jobs and with attending committee meetings, that they had really lost contact with their children, hardly knew them.

THE EMPHASIS ON MATERIAL THINGS

An overlapping problem is excessive materialism. People have to be materialistic in any society to keep from starving. But in most parts of the world, spiritual values hold materialism in check. It was different in my youth; my mother shamed me into turning down a summer job during college because it was too cushy.

In many countries, the family is of enormous importance. A child grows up feeling a great obligation to the family and pride that he is nearly old enough and wise enough to participate in the family business. Geoffrey Gorer, the English anthropologist, said years ago that in other parts of the world a father says to his boy: "Son, ours is a great family. We have given you good food, and good clothes, a good education, now it is up to you to prove that you're worthy of the family." In America this is turned upside down. A father says to his boy: "Son, if you don't do better than I have done, I won't think much of you." In other words, the respect goes primarily to the children. I think that children should be learning to respect their parents and their grandparents. In America the best that many grandparents can hope for, in a society that changes so rapidly, is to be tolerated.

RELIGION

In many other parts of the world and in earlier America, religion has been a compelling force. Children grow up believing that they are in the world to do the Lord's work and that the Lord will give them guidance all day, all year long. We still have a lot of people who go to church, but I don't think many of them are looking to God for guidance all day. We lose a lot if we feel we are all alone and there are no beliefs to stabilize us and give us conviction.

TOLERANCE OF VIOLENCE

We are by far the most violent country in the world as far as I know. A gun control organization a few years ago compared murders with handguns in the United States and in other similar countries. Their figures showed that no other nation had as many as forty deaths from handguns per year; Britain had eight. Do you know what the figure was for the United States? Eleven-thousand-five-hundred-twenty-two. Most of these murders are committed against family members or lovers. Our figures for rape, wife abuse, and child abuse are also shockingly high. These comparisons give an idea of the seething tensions in many families here, and also of the lack of control.

I put part of the blame for violence on television and movies. The average American child by age eighteen has watched eighteen thousand murders on television. Combine that with psychological studies that have shown that every time a child or an adult watches violence, it desensitizes and brutalizes, to a slight degree. But even if this is only to a tiny degree, by the time you multiply that by eighteen thousand, you get a lot of brutalization. It's not that viewing turns a well-loved child into a thug, but everyone is moved in the direction of insensitivity and brutality.

SEXUALITY AND SPIRITUALISM

There has been a coarsening of many people's attitude toward sexuality. It has become despiritualized. Partly, this too has been a result of movies and television. And partly it has been an unintended result of the effort of the sex education movement to remove the fear and shame that used to be a powerful aspect of children's (and adults') attitude toward sex. The movement has emphasized the naturalness of sex and presented it primarily in anatomical terms. This has been a great improvement over the fear and shame of the olden days.

But it neglected in most explanations to emphasize that sexuality is potentially as much spiritual and idealistic as it is physical, that it included the dedication of husbands and wives to each other, their desire to raise fine children and their respect for their children. Sex education leaves out the role of sexuality as an inspiration for poets, writers, composers, architects, painters, sculptors, inventors. It is part of the appreciation as well as the creation of these arts. Children need to hear these spiritual aspects of sexuality just as much as they hear about the anatomy.

A thirteen-year-old told me, "Sex is a perfectly normal instinct, meant to be enjoyed." That's correct as far as it goes. But human beings write poetry, compose music, paint pictures and design beautiful buildings, all of which are partly derived from sublimated, idealized sexuality, and none of which rabbits (who also have an "instinct" for sex) are able to do. I believe that the loss of the spiritual, idealistic side of sex is part of the reason for the great increase in teenage pregnancies, for the coarse view of sexuality in many people, in movies and on television, and for the epidemic of divorce.

Our species has to have beliefs—spiritual beliefs in the broad meaning of spirituality—especially during a transitional stage like the end of adolescence and the beginning of young adulthood. There are quite a few young people today who weren't raised with any deep beliefs and who don't see anything to believe in. That leaves some of them quite frightened, wanting to clutch at anything. As a result of uncertainty and an absence of beliefs, teen suicides have quadrupled in the past twenty years.

CAUSE FOR OPTIMISM

I sometimes ask myself if there isn't something good that's happening in our society. I have two items to be glad about. One is that people are marrying later, on the average. That's good because, though early marriages can be very successful, the younger you marry the more the statistics for success are against you. The other good thing is that people are having children a little later in life. It used to be thought that you ought to have your children when you are young and resilient. Studies have shown that it is the other way around, that there is a good deal of intolerance of children by some young parents. It is the more mature parents, in their late twenties and thirties, who are on the average more understanding and more successful in managing their children. Of course, many younger parents, with support from their families and communities, can raise emotionally healthy children.

I believe that most of our serious problems could be cured, provided that people become more sharply aware of them and of what is needed, and then work actively on the solutions. I say this because of my own experience. For example, I witnessed a real revolution in infant feeding. It resulted primarily from mothers' protests against old-fashioned rules. So pediatric teachings were changed—from rigidity to flexibility in schedules, from urging or forcing in giving foods to following the baby's lead, and in encouraging breast feeding which had almost disappeared.

Political activity also brings about change when there is active participation in a cause you believe in. Though the Vietnam war, for example, dragged on for eight long years because of the determination of two presidents, abetted by the congressional hawks, it was primarily the persistent pressure of a large, organized peace movement that turned public and congressional opinion around, caused Lyndon Johnson to retire from the presidency, and finally brought the war to an end.

AN IDEAL OF SERVICE

I think first that we need to give our children an ideal of service in life; second that parents should be more politically discriminating and active to secure for our children the urgent necessities that we can't provide at home.

I believe that we should raise children not with an emphasis on getting ahead, but primarily to serve, to be helpful, to be cooperative, to be polite, to be kind, to be loving. I don't mean preaching to them or scolding them, because I have a dim view of both. It is a matter of giving them opportunities from the age of two, to be helpful.

We can show our appreciation to the two-year-old who helps put the forks and spoons on the table or brings them back to the kitchen. "You did it so nicely; pretty soon you will be able to put the plates on the table too." It's exciting to a two- and three-year-old to hear that they are making progress on the way to becoming adults.

By five and six years of age children can and should, I feel, have regular simple duties at home and be expected to be polite to their parents and the parents' friends. I remember that my brother and sisters and I were taught by eight years to wash our own clothes in a tub during summer vacations (I don't know how clean we got them) and to pick up our rooms at home.

By nine or ten years, children might be expected to vacuum their rooms and make their beds. By twelve they can mow the lawn, rake the leaves, and wash the car, preferably with the participation of a parent, to tactfully keep them from forgetting.

What should be the connection between chores and allowance? Some parents require that certain chores be completed in order to earn an allowance. Other parents do not connect the two. Either way works. I don't think of this as a crucial matter. But I do feel that children should expect to be called on for extra help when there are minor family crises, without being paid for it. It should be part of being a member of the family.

All teenagers, I feel, should be doing some kind of community service like helping to tutor younger children at school who are having trouble with their lessons, or working in hospitals and other children's institutions, not just to be helpful but to see how many children are deprived or suffering, and how kindliness helps.

One thing that strikes me dramatically among teenagers is the difference between those who are cordial when introduced to an adult friend of their parents, and those who appear bored or hostile (perhaps it's only appearance) and say not a word. I realize that adolescents may be naturally moody, self-conscious, hardly aware that they are making some kind of impression on others. But I think that their parents should tactfully make them aware of the attractive or unattractive impressions they make.

In all these examples of how children can be helpful and polite, I want to emphasize that I don't think parents can get good results from scolding. They should show firmness and confidence toward their children from an early age while tipping them off on how to make a good impression on the world. Best of all is when the parents themselves demonstrate consistent cordiality to each other and to their children.

I believe that to cut down on competitiveness we ought to get rid of all grades in school and in colleges. That idea is shocking to so many people, but I happened to teach in a medical school that has successfully gotten rid of grades. If you can get rid of grades in medical school you certainly ought to be able to get rid of grades in elementary school and high school. I think grades mislead children and they mislead teachers. They give children the idea that if they get higher grades they've become that much wiser which isn't necessarily true at all. It seems to me as a teacher that what is necessary for good grades is first to have a good memory, and secondly to accept compliantly what the teacher says. I think also that good grades mislead teachers into thinking that the children who get higher grades are wiser or will be more successful. I believe that what should be emphasized in school are such matters as initiative, ability to make up your own mind, a sense of responsibility, and encouragement of creativity. I believe that we shouldn't have any physical punishment or humiliation of children. That is going to take a lot of doing in the United States, where a large proportion of parents believe that you can't bring up a child properly without spanking him from time to time. This is simply not true as I am sure many of you have found out. I've known dozens and dozens of families where the children were not only never punished, they were never humiliated and yet they were as polite and cooperative as you could possibly wish. What you have to do with children in many ways is treat them from early childhood the way you treat adults. It is a matter of showing them respect, asking for their cooperation, and asking for their respect for you too.

The reason that I was mealymouthed about physical

punishment in early editions of *Baby and Child Care* was knowing that so many parents believe punishment is absolutely essential, and believing strongly myself that a professional person shouldn't criticize parents and say, "You don't know how to raise your children. I know how and I'll tell you." But now that I have gotten more experience, I dare to say that I believe that it is better to bring up children feeling that they want to behave because they love their parents and they want to be loved by their parents, rather than because they fear punishment.

Needless to say I am violently opposed to children watching violence on television and in movies. The same goes for crude, loveless sex. I think that, to be more constructive about it, parents ought to be putting pressure on advertisers, on the local station and on the networks. "Give our children something good to watch on television." It is the greatest educational force that has ever been invented. It is a shame that it is being used to foster violence and to sell children sugar-coated cereals that undermine their nutrition and rot their teeth. All other industrial countries that I know of have programs for children. We have a couple of programs for preschool children but there are none for older children. This forces them to entertain themselves with television programs that give emphasis to violence or trash.

The other vital area in which we ought to make more progress is in political activity in support of children's causes. There are contradictory attitudes here among American parents. They are, as a rule, generous to a fault in providing, for their own children, music and dancing lessons, tooth straightening, and sacks of fine playthings for holidays and birthdays. But when it comes to establishing services for all children through political activity—health care for all, high quality day care for all who need it, challenging schools especially for children growing up in deprived neighborhoods, decent housing for all, rescue facilities for neglected and abused children—Americans show much less concern and political activity than citizens in many other developed countries. Social and educational programs for children and families in Scandinavian countries are one example.

In fact, as you know, only half of eligible American citizens bother to vote at all. And some of those who do vote seem to me to vote for the candidate with the pleasanter smile rather than the one who will work hardest for the things that families need. If you feel strongly about an issue that the local candidates seem to be ignoring, you can organize a political meeting at a club or school or church at which local candidates are invited to speak. If the candidates for Senate, the House, or local office seem equally unresponsive on your vital issue, you can help to organize backing for a challenger in the nominating election. Nothing gets an office holder's attention better than to hear that he or she will be challenged for the nomination.

After a candidate has been elected, opportunities for further political activity open up in other directions. Letter-writing always has an impact, as all elected officials agree. You can write every time you get hot under the collar—once a month if it's called for. You can form a small committee and lobby the official at his post or when he next visits his local office. You can demonstrate with signs in front of his office. You can write letters to the editor of your paper. Civil disobedience is not everyone's choice of political action, but it attracts ten times as much media attention as a polite demonstration, especially if well-known citizens and members of the clergy participate.

The important thing is not which political activity you engage in—as long as it suits your beliefs and feelings—but how often and how persistently you keep it up.

Throughout childhood children will be watching their parents and, except during adolescence, trying to pattern themselves after their parents. That does not mean that parents have to be perfect, but that they should respect each other and the children, let their spiritual values show, not only in expressing their opinions at the dinner table but in the attitudes and behavior toward family and friends. Also toward other groups in the town, nation, and the world. The parents' tolerance, generosity, affection, and their working for a better world are important for the children to see. But most important of all is the parents' expression of love for the children, not only in words but in occasional spontaneous hugs.

Am I an optimist or a pessimist? I'm both, depending on whether parents rise to the challenges or not. If they do we can make a better society.

Children and Religion

I believe all children are born with the capacity and the inclination to be spiritual and religious beings. It starts with their profound love for their parents in early childhood. It's a dependent love; they feel anxious when they are separated from their parents. They admire them to an exaggerated quite unrealistic degree; they think their parents are the most beautiful, wise, powerful people in the world. They want to help their parents, give them presents. They want to grow up to be like them and they spend a lot of time imitating them. They fear their parents' disapproval. They accept God on their parents' say-so. He seems like a grandfather, predominantly approving or disapproving depending on the parents' general attitude.

When children get to be six and seven years old, they outgrow some of their slavish drive to be exactly like their parents. They pay more attention to other boys and girls and want to be like them. They get interested in who the authorities outside the family are: the police, the mayor, the president, and God. In a religious family—and a majority of families are at least nominally religious—they hear the love, the respect, and the awe that their parents, clergyman, and Sunday-school teachers feel for God. So a lot of the feelings that younger children felt for their parents are now transferred to God. Their feeling for God is predominantly respect for his authority rather than a personal love. They get interested in such matters as heaven and hell and why their parents are or are not religious.

In families in which the parents have little love to give and no religious devotion to teach, the children are unlikely to show much in the way of spiritual qualities or religious beliefs.

For adolescents the situation becomes more complex. They are at a stage when their feelings for other people become intense. They may develop a crush on an adult—one whom they know or a distant entertainer. They fall in love with another boy or girl. Some become deeply religious. Others, feeling the common impulse to rebel against their parents, may object to attending their parents' church or synagogue. In later years they may come back to religion or remain agnostics or atheists, partly depending on whether they have come around to a comfortable relationship with their parents.

I consider fortunate the children born into a family that adheres to a specific religion or a firm set of moral standards. These give them a comforting framework, explains life's mysteries, shows them exactly what their society and their religion expects of them. If their family's religion or spiritual values teach love, generosity, tolerance, and understanding, these qualities will foster their maturity, their acceptance of others, their contribution to the happiness of others and themselves. I say "if" because studies show that membership in some churches fosters intolerance and unfriendliness toward those belonging to another church or no church.

I believe that it is beneficial for children in the middle and the adolescent years to attend Sunday school, as part of their general education, to learn the Bible stories and the commonly sung hymns; to learn what Christians, Jews, and Moslems mean by God, sin, salvation, and forgiveness; to think about their own naturally evolving beliefs, and, if they come to join a church or synagogue, to feel part of a religious movement that has existed for hundreds of years and involved millions of people. I believe that parents should strongly encourage their children to attend Sunday school as part of their education even if the parents are not church members or believers at all.

Children up to the age of adolescence are not likely to object to going to church or temple with their parents, to a Sunday school that their parents have selected or that their friends attend.

In adolescence, the parents may be quite firm that their child attend their church or synagogue, if they have that kind of control or if their child is of a compliant nature. If the child is rebellious, I'd say it was a mistake for the parents to try to dictate. It would be more likely to make the child antireligious during adolescence.

At the beginning of this discussion, I spoke of children being inclined to be religious and spiritual. I meant that when the parents have no religious affiliation or belief, but have strong spiritual drives—in the sense of devoted love of each other and of their children, honesty with their associates, tolerance of those who are different, generosity toward those who are unfortunate—their children will naturally pick up these spiritual attitudes in early childhood through their love, admiration, and identification with their parents. In middle childhood they will turn more to their friends but seek out friends raised with the same ideals as themselves. In adolescence they will turn even more to admired models outside the family in the sense of hero worship or crushes on adults.

Are there values in prayer? I would say definitely yes in adolescence when the child knows what she is saying to God, especially if she has composed the prayer. She is thinking about her anxieties, her guilt, her needs; prayer will help her to understand herself and she will feel closer to God and comforted by the experience.

Causes for Children

Should parents try to involve their children in the solution of local and world problems? There is a wide variety, of course: The foreign and home missions that children hear about in church and Sunday school. There are many environmental dangers, such as acid rain, oil spills, smog, the warming of the earth that results in the "greenhouse effect" from carbon monoxide, and the accumulation of trash and toxins. There are the visible social ills of homelessness, poverty, and dilapidated housing. There are the TV pictures of starving adults and children in some foreign countries and the reports of hunger and malnutrition in our own land. Television shows wars raging in the Middle East, in Africa, in Southeast Asia. The AIDS epidemic is gathering speed around the world and involving babies. Drug abuse is raging particularly among the poor and is doing serious damage to thousands of children.

Our children see these scourges on television news, see pictures in the newspapers, hear discussion by their parents and by other children. Some older children enjoy scaring younger children with true or distorted stories. So there is no way to keep children in ignorance. They show that they have been affected by the worried questions they ask. We learned from questionnaires given to school-age children in the 1960s that many more children than parents are worried about a nuclear war. Children suffer in sympathy with victims and they worry about becoming victims themselves.

I believe that it's wise for parents to bring out into the open and discuss with their children the concerns that children show by their direct or indirect questions. The parents should be able to straighten out the exaggerated and often distorted ideas that children acquire. I don't think it's wise to tell young children about tragedies of which they are not yet aware.

Parents should be able to show children that there are solutions or partial solutions to most of the world's problems. This helps children to cope better with their anxieties. For anxiety is given to us to spur us to action and the action decreases the anxiety to a greater or lesser degree. The main point is not so much to protect children from being excessively disturbed by the world's problems but to go further and give them positive attitudes about possible solutions.

I believe that parents and teachers should feel a responsibility to build into children's characters a life-long conviction that they are in this world not merely to fulfill themselves but to help make the world a better place, whether they will go into one of the so-called helping occupations—teaching, health care, or social work—or into business or industry. I say this because I believe that our country and our world are in great peril, which is getting worse rather than better. The economy is deteriorating, the middle and working classes are getting poorer. Homelessness is increasing. More mothers have to work and some of their children are being deprived of security because of the scarcity of high-quality day care. Drug use is increasing. So is teenage pregnancy. Discrimination festers. Murder within the family and both spousal abuse and child abuse are shockingly high. Our world cannot be saved unless the coming generations are not only aware and concerned about the problems but are dedicated to helping to solve them throughout their lifetimes.

The most fundamental way to orient children to helping solve the country's problems is for their parents to set an example. It's in the three- to six-year-old period that children are watching their parents intently—imitating their way of talking and walking, their daily activities, and taking on their interests as far as they can understand them. In the middle years of childhood, from seven to about twelve years old, they are not as inclined to imitate their parents exactly, but they are still influenced strongly by their parents' fundamental beliefs. In adolescence, feelings become much more intense. They want to live up to the expectations of their friends and be accepted by them. So they are likely to be critical or rebellious about some of their parents' beliefs and standards. But in their twenties, they often swing back in the general direction of their parents' ideals though they may well differ in the details.

In all these various periods of childhood, parents should feel free to talk about their causes when chatting with their children. But they would be wise not to speak as if they expect their adolescents to agree with them, not to speak as if they think they are wiser in their opinions because they are older. Teenagers are often interested in their parents' views, though they usually avoid revealing this. They resent any effort by their parents to impose their views on them, to be talked to in a condescending manner or to be talked at too long. For if parents are tactless in such matters, it gets adolescents' backs up, pushes their views in the opposite direction, and delays or prevents their swinging around to their parents' position in their twenties.

It's the parents' actions that affect children more than words. For example, taking their voting responsibilities seriously, writing letters, sending an E-mail or telephoning the president, their senators, their representative, writing letters to the editor of the local newspaper, and going with a group to lobby at the local office of senators and representatives when those officers come to town.

I think it is reassuring and worthwhile for young children, especially if they are anxious about some threat to health or safety, to join their parents in writing a letter to the president, their senators, their representative, the governor, the mayor, whoever may be appropriate, if this appeals to them. It gives them the conviction that they are doing something that will really help and I believe it will. A child's letter is apt to sound more sincere and persuasive than an adult's letter. If the parents are activists and are involved in marching or picketing or demonstrating, and a child wants to join them, I think it's good for the child's anxiety, good for her future effectiveness as a citizen, and good for the country. However some school-age children and many adolescents are shy about doing anything unconventional in public, and I wouldn't put the slightest pressure on any child who hesitated or wasn't eager.

Fostering the right spirit should begin early. In influencing children to be concerned, to be generous, to be idealistic, don't forget to expect them to be helpful at home (for example, helping to set the table beginning at two years old) and in the neighborhood (volunteering in hospitals and other local institutions) as they enter adolescence.

Violence in the News, Movies, and on Television

Children may see all manners of horrors in the newspaper and on television news. A plane crashes and the bodies of children and adults are strewn on the ground. An insane man opens fire in a crowded restaurant, killing adults and children. Another insane man shoots children in their classroom.

You can expect quite a range of responses to the news of such tragedies from different children, depending on age and sensitivity. School-age children from about six to twelve years old are generally more toughened by knowledge of what goes on in the world. They are naturally more interested in violent comics and games than younger children and therefore somewhat less likely to be upset.

Adolescents are, of course, more familiar still with the seamy sides of life and furthermore, take pride in their sophistication. So, even if they are at first inwardly shocked by some distressing event, they quickly try to fit it into their previous picture of the world and act as if they had known about such things all along.

By contrast, children under six years old tend to be much more sensitive. They know little of what goes on in the world outside their family, so they have little basis for evaluating an unusual experience. Young children get the full impact of a disturbing occurrence from their raw feelings; they have no defenses. And more than children of an older age, they immediately apply anything fearsome that happens to someone else to themselves. I remember vividly how one of my sons at the age of four years gazed horrified at a newspaper photograph of a man's head protruding from an old-fashioned iron lung, while I tried to reassure him by explaining that the man couldn't breathe for himself so this machine breathed for him. Suddenly my son grabbed his throat in terror and whispered hoarsely, "I can't breathe!"

Young children, because of their innocence and the strength of their imagination, can be disturbed by animated cartoons of animals as much as by scenes of real-life humans.

In addition to the factor of age, there is the factor of individual sensitivity. Doctors now call this *temperament*—the way our brain influences our emotions when faced with new situations. I've known a few children who were on the edge of fearfulness even during the first year of life—they had a slightly apprehensive expression even when their lives appeared to me to be going smoothly. They quickly became panicky when they fell down or when barked at by a dog. At three years old, they are apt to be scared of the dark or of unfamiliar people. These overly sensitive, timid and fearful children are particularly likely to be disturbed by violence on television news. At the opposite extreme is the young child who walks right up to strange people, strange animals, and strange, noisy machines with an expression of happy curiosity.

A few children in middle childhood and even in

adolescence are easily upset. A movie about a monster may worry them for weeks. If they temporarily lose a parent in a crowd, they may go to pieces and become panicky. Hearing about a kidnapping on television makes them fear the same fate; they may suspect that any slightly unusual man they see in the street is a kidnapper.

Is there harm in children watching violence, whether or not they are unusually sensitive? I believe we have definite evidence that there are two kinds of harm. The first is that, among the most fearful children, fearfulness will be increased and made longer lasting when they are frightened by external events or scenes or stories. The second harm is that many of the majority of children, who have a more neutral temperament, will be desensitized to violence. They will come to feel that it isn't bad, that it's just a normal part of life. This gives them moral permission to get into fights and to beat up members of their family. Those children brought up without much in the way of standards or ideals can be influenced by television brutality to commit violent crimes, including murder.

How can you prevent your children from being disturbed by television violence, either in the news or in dramatic programs? If it's a dramatic program with a lot of continuing violence, you can and should, I believe, matter-of-factly forbid your children to watch such programs, and check up every few days to make sure your rule is being followed. Since you never know when violence will crop up in television news, I think that young and school-age children should be forbidden to watch news programs, unless some program is a special documentary that you feel will be educational and devoid of brutality.

But, you may object, shouldn't children be encouraged to follow the news? I believe that adolescents should be encouraged, but that few under that age will be trying to learn constructively about the nation and the world from television news. If you have school-age children who do seem to be genuinely interested, you can compromise by having children and parents watch the news together. Then if brutal stories crop up, you can take away some of the horror by explaining, for instance, that it is only insane parents who do cruel things to their children. That's stretching the exact meaning of insane, but it is a direct way of making clear that normal parents don't suddenly attack their children.

If my child asked whether there was any chance he might be attacked by a relative, I wouldn't hesitate to say, calmly, "No. No chance at all."

When children have been disturbed by any kind of horror, the best thing that parents can do is encourage them to talk about what they've seen, what they think caused it, what they are worrying about for themselves. It's better in this way to explore children's own fantasies and fears first, so that you'll know how to go about reassuring them. I say this because kind parents usually have the impulse to reassure quickly, when they have only a vague general idea of what the fear is. This kind of hasty reassurance often misses the target, and leaves the child still worrying about his particular fear that hasn't been addressed yet. It's hard for adults to imagine what children's true worries are, because they may be so weird.

I recall a study about what worried children, who were in the hospital for tonsillectomy, think about. A number assumed that the operation was punishment for wrongdoing—that they had caught too many sore throats because they hadn't worn their gloves or coats or galoshes in bad weather. A child who had been moved to a different room after admission to the hospital was in despair because she assumed her parents wouldn't be able to find her when it was time to go home. A boy thought that during a tonsillectomy the surgeon cut the throat from ear to ear, tipped the head back like the lid on a coffeepot, and reached into the wound to cut out the tonsils. In such cases, the parent who offers general reassurances without first finding out the child's specific fears would not be much help.

One of the harms of conflict in television news is that children tend to identify with any group of people who seem to be the victims in a confrontation, even if there is no explicit brutality shown—when the police, for instance, are controlling a crowd in the street during a political demonstration or when striking women factory workers are picketing and the police are trying to control them. So "law and order" can seem violent.

It has been calculated that three quarters of children's viewing of television is in "prime time" so that is the time for you to be vigilant about what your children are watching. Why do many parents allow their children to watch violence not only on television but in the movies as well? I ask the question because I believe that such viewing experiences are harmful for children.

Fifty years ago, when I first began pediatric practice, I didn't have the same attitude. When a mother opposed to violence would express her worry that playing with guns and listening to radio violence (there was no television then) might turn her young son into a insensitive or cruel person, I would pooh-pooh the connection. I'd explain that playing at violence is a normal stage of development in the three- to twelve-year-old period.

What first made me reverse my opinion, nearly thirty years ago, was the comment of an experienced, mature nursery school teacher who told me that soon after *The Three Stooges* program became popular, the children began to bop each other without provocation. When she would protest to a child who had just hit another child that the victim had done nothing to justify this, the hitter wouldn't show any regret or concern. He would say indignantly, "That's what the Three Stooges do." This revealed to me, suddenly and chillingly, that children—especially young children—will accept and pattern themselves after violent behavior just as readily as after ideal behavior. Whatever adults do is okay!

Another example of violence learned in childhood is demonstrated in recent investigations of families in which there is cruel abuse of children. In a great majority of cases, the abusing parents themselves had been abused in their childhood and that was when they came to accept abuse as permissible parental behavior.

In recent years there have been a number of psychological studies and observations that prove without any doubt that watching violence has a desensitizing and a brutalizing effect. By desensitizing, I mean that individuals brought up in compassionate and good-natured families will at first be shocked and horrified when they see one person do violence to another. But if they continue to see it regularly, they will gradually get over the horror and take it for granted. It's like becoming emotionally numb to repeated exposures to violence.

It has been calculated that the average American child has seen eighteen thousand murders on television before reaching adulthood. That will produce a lot of desensitization and brutalization of feelings, in the long run. This does not mean that a child brought up in a kind family will be turned into a thug by watching violence on film and on television. But everyone, tough or gentle, will be moved bit by bit, in the direction of insensitivity and harshness.

I believe that it is particularly unfortunate for American children to be raised with a tolerance for violence. For as a nation, we already have shockingly high figures for murder within the family, for rape, for wife abuse, and for child abuse, probably the highest in the world. Yet we are surely creating more and more such cruelty by television violence.

Under these circumstances, I think it is irresponsible and provocative for television and movie producers to be putting out so many films that exalt violence. A current example that distresses me is the series about Rambo, a bully who goes around imposing his will on others through muscular might and fiendish weapons, in a manner which will appeal to boys.

There has been a thorough analysis of studies on the effects of television violence, and the conclusion of these studies was that watching violence is definitely harmful to children. The Surgeon General of the Public Health Service issued a similar conclusion.

There must be reasons why so many parents continue to let their children watch violence in spite of the conclusive evidence of harm. Probably some parents have not heard of these studies. Others may be skeptical about the harm since they see no observable differences in their children's behavior from one day to the next. This is because the desensitization and emotional numbing come gradually.

But the largest number, I suspect, simply shrink back from the prospect of the chore it would be to carefully supervise their children's television viewing—not just today and next week but for the endless arguments that children will put up when they want some privilege or possession that their parents are reluctant to give them. They try to grind their parents down if the parents show any evidence of hesitancy.

Now we should get down to asking how parents can get less harmful television programs and movies for their children. They should put the pressure on local television stations and movie theaters, on networks, on advertisers, not just to cut out the violence but to provide children with challenging, constructive programs and movies. All other modern nations provide good programs for children of various ages, and there is no reason why the world's richest nation shouldn't do at least as well. There could be travel films that show how people live in other parts of the world, nature films, science films, adventure films. They can be just as fascinating as violence.

In calling on station managers and movie house managers, and in writing to networks and advertisers, it's wasteful to go it alone. Organize a committee of at least a couple of dozen people, and come up with a serious name that describes your project. Some of the organizations you can write to are:

National Coalition on Television Violence
5132 Newport Avenue, Bethesda, MD 20816
www.nctvv.org

Action for Children's Television
20 University Road, Cambridge, MA 02138
(617) 876-6620

Media Action Research Center (MARC)
475 Riverside Drive, Suite 1070
New York, NY 10015
(212) 865-6690

The Motion Picture Association of America
1600 I Street, NW
Washington, DC 20006
(202) 293-1966

The Advertising Council
825 Third Avenue
New York, NY 10022
(212) 758-0400

Federal Communications Commission
Chief of Complaints—Mass Media Bureau
1919 M Street, NW
Washington, DC 20554

American Broadcasting Company (ABC)
Audience Information
1330 Avenue of the Americas
New York, NY 10019
(212) 887-7777

Cable Network News (CNN)
Public Information
1 CNN Center
P.O. Box 105366
Atlanta, GA 30374-0166
(404) 827-1500

Columbia Broadcasting System (CBS)
Entertainment Division

51 West 52nd Street
New York, NY 10019
(212) 975-4321

National Broadcasting Company (NBC)
Audience Services
30 Rockefeller Plaza
New York, NY 10020
(212) 664-4444

Meanwhile, what should parents do about the programs that exist today? They should absolutely forbid
their children, I believe, to watch programs that deal in
violence, brutality, and explicit, loveless sex. This
means, first of all, that parents must keep a sharp eye
on what their children are watching. Secondly, they
must really mean it when they forbid a certain program. It won't work if they forbid it when they think of
it on Monday or Wednesday but fail to notice that the
children have gone back to it on Tuesday, Thursday,
and Friday—or notice but feel too tired to argue.

I'm firmly convinced that if parents feel strongly that
something is bad for their children they can make a
prohibition stick. It's when they are uncertain and vac-
illating that children get the message that arguments or
persistence or sneakiness will work often enough to be
well worth a try.

What about the children who know that their parents are apt to be tied up—with supper preparation, for
instance—at the time some of the forbidden programs

come on and so disobey; or the children who manage to be visiting friends each day when popular programs show; or the "latchkey" children who are not under supervision at crucial hours? I have several answers.

If parents have the respect of their children and good control, their rules should and will generally be obeyed, even when they are not there. But to be sure that their children know that they mean business, the parents should check up occasionally in the middle of supper preparation, for example, or phone the house when they suspect their child may be watching television.

What about the violence in television cartoons, especially all Saturday morning, and the violence in the comics? I would keep a young child—up to the age of six years let's say—from seeing both, because up to that age children are not at all clear about the difference between make-believe and reality; make-believe violence seems as frightening and brutalizing as the real thing.

After the age of about six or seven years, there is somewhat less harm in cartoons and comics because children recognize them as inventions of an artist. But this is not to say that they are good for children to see. They are still desensitizing in the sense that they make brutality to cartoon animals and to comic-strip humans a laughing matter rather than something shocking.

Even after the age of six years, I'd urge parents to prohibit movies and television programs showing human actors committing violence on others—strangling, smashing a person in the face, knocking him unconscious, pushing him off a height, shooting him in the head—for they are so skillfully acted that it's impossible not to react to them with horror at first, and then gradually to take them for granted as standard human behavior.

2

Families

The Changing Family

I feel that the importance of the American family is being eroded in small, subtle or obvious ways. The demands of the workplace and of schools, the excessive mobility of our society, the materialism of our beliefs, the weakening of religious beliefs—these are just a few of the changes tugging at the bonds that connect the generations. For instance, the simple ceremony of sitting down to eat dinner together has been abandoned in many families; overworked fathers and mothers tend to lose contact with their children and with each other; and family members are busy with so many outside activities that they don't have time for one another. Because of this, I worry that children are feeling less connected to their parents and, ultimately, less self-assured.

The causes of this shift are complex, but I think the main reason is that many American parents take their work more seriously than their families. And this, I believe, is where we need to change our thinking. As parents, we have to decide that family comes first and to make it clear to our children that they are more important than anything else in our lives.

Even friendships, neighborhood activities, and cultural interests should take higher priority than most jobs, because these are what humanize us and show our children what matters most. I don't want to get in an argument about whether or not Einstein's work should have been his first priority, but I am suggesting that during the child-rearing years, parents shift their career into the background and bring the family into the foreground. This may be easy for me to say, but I think parents should make whatever sacrifices are necessary for that to happen—whether it means getting by on less income for several years or temporarily postponing certain aims and pursuits.

If parents do make financial sacrifices to be at home with their children, they should be offered subsidies—from government or from their employers. It's crazy for parents who prefer to care for their children to pay someone else to do it. Of course, most of us still have to work. And a serious challenge for most working parents is how to find the best care for their children during working hours.

High-quality day care is expensive and hard to find. Child-care workers are miserably paid, and make their own sacrifices to go into those occupations. We should be raising their salaries, but families on modest incomes just can't afford to pay more for child care. It's going to have to be paid for by the government and industry, as it is in a majority of European countries.

We need to acknowledge, as a nation, that poor-quality day care is a serious deprivation, and a child will never completely outgrow the loss of warmhearted and understanding care. I think we're going to pay seriously in future generations for the lack of good day care that's being provided today. We're going to pay for it in emotional insecurity and in crime. We need day-care workers who are carefully selected and thoroughly trained in child development. These workers and professionals need to know that what children need most isn't policing and disciplining, but stimulation and kindness. We want to attract people to go into day care primarily because they love children.

As a pediatrician during the past sixty-five years, I've seen far-reaching changes in the American family. One of the biggest changes is that nearly 25 percent of American families now live in what would have been considered "nontraditional" households sixty-five years ago, including single divorced parents, single unmarried parents, stepfamilies, unmarried partners, gay and lesbian partners, and just about any configuration you can think of.

A 1950s-style household has been the standard family pattern for so long that many of us still find it hard to accept that the nuclear family is now only one type of arrangement. People talk about family values and somehow that has been translated into the traditional nuclear family. The makeup of a family is less important than the values and ways of child-rearing that parents bring to their children. Three recent trends will illustrate the effects of change on all families regardless of their composition.

HESITANCY

What I'd call "parental hesitancy" has become the most common problem in raising children. Many parents show a lack of firmness in dealing with their children. Equally important, they're reluctant to discuss and clarify their principles about crucial topics such as human relations and important aims in life.

To some parents, it seems that discipline is either black or white. Either you've got to be a disagreeable dominating boss, or the child takes over. But there are other possibilities. To get a child to cooperate, you don't need to be rigid, or severe, or use physical punishment. You can be friendly and understanding and still be the one who's wise enough to know that even if your child argues, that doesn't change the fact that it's bedtime or mealtime. Firmness is simply knowing what you consider good for your child and presenting that message consistently. A parent should provide clear leadership—the child needs to know what the parent expects.

SEX EDUCATION

When it comes to educating children about sex, the parents' role has become even more difficult. In the move to be more open about answering their children's questions, many parents are unclear about how to convey their values. And children, who hear and see so much in the media, aren't always sure who or what to believe. I think it's great that sex can be talked about and that parents are no longer scaring their children or making them guilty. But I believe that in the swing from instilling guilt to teaching that sex is a natural, wholesome topic, we've turned it into merely an anatomy or physiology lesson. While the purely physical aspects alone may describe sex for rabbits, for human beings sexuality is an incredibly subtle, elaborate, and powerful matter.

From the earliest ages, parents should try to keep the lines of communication open about sex, and let their child know that questions are encouraged. Mothers and fathers should talk not only about physiology, but also about how sex is a very intense relationship. It's one of the main reasons people decide to get married and raise fine children. The most important aspect of sex is its contribution to our emotional, cultural, and spiritual life, so when talking to our children, the strongest emphasis should be on mutual love, dedication, and intense child-parent relations.

SCIENCE REPLACES SPIRITUALITY

Just as important as developing children's physical health is developing their spiritual values and sense of idealism. When I use the word "spirituality," I'm talking not only about religion but about very simple things like service to others, kindliness, loyalty, and lovingness, qualities that are often underemphasized in our materialistic culture today.

One of the main reasons for the weakness of idealism and spiritual values today is that over the past couple of centuries science has replaced religion in the minds of many people. They have accepted science as a substitute for religion and spirituality. But they have forgotten that science has never dealt in a forthright way with the soul. Science is materialistic.

When I was a young adult I thought that beliefs were less important than being a decent, well-educated person. I no longer feel that way. We are a believing species. We must believe in a religion or in other spiritual attitudes, or we find that we put materialism first.

MAKING A DIFFERENCE

Children are now often brought up to believe that they're in the world only to get ahead. I've heard parents say, in effect, to their children, "Don't worry about politics, don't worry about war and peace, don't get so concerned about the meaning of life. Your job is to make money and to get ahead." One result of all this is that we tend to forget about the needs of others. We aren't as concerned about the welfare of all children or about other public issues.

In this country's revolutionary era, our citizens believed that the right to decide their own destiny was worth fighting for. Nowadays, fewer than half the eligible voters go to the polls on election day. I find this sad and alarming. If this country had fewer problems, if everybody had a job and health care and an inspiring education, I could perhaps understand it. But that's not the case.

I don't think it requires another revolution for America to once again think of the collective good of all its citizens. But both parents and educators need to hammer home the message about the importance of getting involved, of voting, of caring for others, of giving. Such lessons are easily taught by example at home. Our children need to learn early that their opinions will count increasingly. Just taking a child's concerns seriously lets her know that others value her.

And if a child feels valued herself, in turn, she is more likely to value others. By developing in her a strong sense of self—in combination with seeing her own parents involved in school, neighborhood fundraisers, charities, local elections—she is likely to be far more caring and giving and helping toward others. And, finally, children should be reminded by their parents' example that it's not what you have that's important, it's what you do for others.

Early or Late Childbearing

Many years ago when I started my pediatric practice, I heard mothers agree, "It's good to have your children when you are young, energetic, closer to them in age." This sounded sensible, and I'd had insufficient contrary experience to doubt it, for most of the mothers I'd met in my early years in pediatric practice were in their twenties.

Then, about thirty years ago I read a book based on an extensive study of family relationships. One of the chapters concerned this very matter of young mothers in late teens or their twenties compared with older mothers in their thirties and early forties, and how the two age groups made out, on the average, in the management of their children. In general, it was the older mothers who had the easier time managing and getting along with their children. A majority of them seemed naturally to be more understanding, more patient, more tolerant; and this accepting attitude in these mothers appeared to produce a generally more cooperative attitude in their children. To put it the other way around, more of the very young mothers tended to be impatient and irritable with their children, and the children in these cases were more likely to be argumentative and uncooperative. I want to emphasize that these are trends from a large study; many young parents do an excellent job in raising their children.

This reminded me of a time when I was teaching medical students in a small clinic that served teenage, unmarried mothers. Many of them spoke critically of their babies' behavior. When we would ask, "How is the baby doing?" they often answered, impatiently, "He's bad." The most common explanation was that he cried a lot. In other words, these mothers made no allowance for the fact that young babies cry often as a way of communicating needs and feelings. They just judged them on a moralistic basis, and judged them rather severely.

This is similar to the hypercritical attitude among some teenage girls toward their preteen brothers. When I would ask such a girl what her younger brother was like, she was apt to make a disgusted sound, "Ugh!," meaning that he still had the crude manners and appearance of the typical ten-year-old boy, with no appreciation of the romantic or elegant aspects of life.

I believe that part of the explanation for the teenager's critical nature—about her baby or of the younger brother—is that she is trying hard to be considered a young woman. But the crying baby or the "crude" brother reminds her subconsciously that she too is still close to childhood. This displeases her and is one of the causes that makes mothers in their late teens and early twenties less understanding and less tolerant of their children than mothers in their thirties.

A principal factor that favors later childbearing these days is that so many young women choose to start their serious work careers right after graduation from high school or college, rather than think first of finding a suitable husband and settling down to raise a family, as they used to in the earlier years of this century. This has been partly the result of the women's liberation movement beginning around 1970. It has emphasized the importance of careers for women, their right to equal pay with men, equal access to the prestigious positions.

The average age for marriage has gone up, too,

probably for several reasons: the increased importance of higher education and careers for women, the efficiency of birth control methods that permit sexual relationships without marriage, and a reaction against the frequent failure of very young marriages. Of course, there were cases of late childbearing before 1970; and there have been cases of very successful early marriage and early childbearing since 1970, despite the predominant trends to the contrary.

Now let's discuss the actual advantages and disadvantages of both late and early childbearing, as mothers have described them to me. The greatest advantage to starting with a career and postponing childbearing is that a woman with serious career ambitions has an opportunity to prove to herself that she has the capabilities to succeed. Back in the first half of this century, girls and young women were often taunted openly that, as females, they didn't have the right temperament to be engineers, or mathematicians, or physicists, or executives. ("Too emotional," was the favorite accusation by insecure men.) Nowadays, most men would be embarrassed to bring up such blatant prejudices, but there are enough residuals of such attitudes floating around to undermine a young woman who lacks self-assurance. To get a strong foundation in a career first may erase these doubts for some women. Furthermore, a good work experience allows the mother to relax and enjoy the baby to the full when she does turn to motherhood. I've been impressed by the intensity of such a mother's delight. She keeps repeating that she had no idea how pleasurable and fulfilling child care would be.

A mother who doesn't have her first child until her thirties has often had earlier opportunities to travel, to experiment, to get involved in hobbies, to take courses. So she doesn't feel she has been robbed of desirable experiences, as she might if she had had children in her early twenties and then went right on to add a job.

A very important reason for later childbearing is that the man and woman have had more of a chance to grow up, in the sense of knowing themselves, knowing and making the adjustment to each other, before taking on the added responsibility of a child. And in most cases the financial situation is more secure.

Are there disadvantages in delayed childbearing? On the physical side, there is the somewhat greater risk of Down's Syndrome (a chromosome disorder associated with developmental delay and disabilities) with increasing age. On the emotional side, there may be an increased temptation to overindulge a late first child, because he's been long awaited or may not be replaceable. But this tendency should be easily recognized and not too difficult to overcome.

The woman who has had some tendency to be a worrier all her life will probably be a more worrisome and overprotective mother if she has her first child near the end of her childbearing period, just as she would if she had difficulty conceiving at any age or had had several miscarriages. All these situations make a mother unusually apprehensive about losing a child who might be difficult or impossible to replace. Such apprehension may lead to too frequent warnings to him about avoiding falls, traffic accidents, colds and other infections, or kidnappers. These warnings have some tendency to make a child either a worrier or, in defiance, a foolish risk-taker. If the parents find that they can't control their worrisomeness, they should be able to get help from a pediatrician, a family social agency, or a mental-health professional.

A few older parents have become too set in their ways to make allowances for a child's normal restlessness, noisiness, or messiness. If parents get the suspicion from self-observation or hints from friends that they are expecting too much conformity from their child, expecting him to be an adult from the start instead of recognizing that he must be a child in a child's world, they can enter him in a preschool class or day-care center from the age of two or three years (not a bad idea for any only child). If that's impossible they should take him to a playground or other gathering place for young children several times a week. The parents can then see how their expectations of behavior stack up against those of other parents, compare other parents' methods, and their child's behavior in a play situation with others. If such efforts are ineffective the parents should be able to get more help from counseling.

Though early or late childbearing may each bring with it particular difficulties (or successes), none of the difficulties is serious enough by itself to override a couple's personal reasons for preferring early or late childbearing. Any sensible couple can make a success of any childbearing schedule that they choose—or that catches them unaware.

The Second Child

In making generalizations about personality and attitudes about the second child, I'm writing about the average second child or the tendencies in most second children. I'm certainly not describing all second children or any one second child. For though there are dramatic contrasts between the personality tendencies of second and first children there are lots of exceptions.

For there are other factors that strongly influence personality aside from place in the family. One is inborn temperament—the behavioral responses of a baby to new situations and stimulations. Studies have shown that babies are born with distinctly different temperaments and that these differences tend to persist for life. One example is a high activity level in one baby compared to the quietness in another. One baby is a bold explorer and experimenter from an early age; another wants to observe, to case the joint, to size up a new situation, before he or she feels ready to venture into it.

Another factor, of course, is the personality of the parent and the parent's attitude toward each child. A warmhearted, enthusiastic mother tends to evoke a hearty responsiveness from her child, while a reserved parent tends to foster reserve in the child. Furthermore, no parent presents exactly the same front to two different children. The kind of parent, let's say it's the father, who wants a son he can roughhouse with may feel slightly frustrated and less outgoing with a son who seems too quiet and gentle. One parent treats a daughter very much the same as a son; another parent treats a daughter and a son entirely differently.

Now we're more ready to deal with the average second child. Let's say it's a boy. First let's think how his world looks to him. He comes into the world in a family that probably consists of two parents and one older child. He soon begins to realize that there are two distinct generations in his family: the parental or adult generation, and the child generation to which he belongs. By the way, I've always been fascinated with the sharp distinction that babies make between children and adults. When another child approaches, even an unknown one, a baby's face is apt to light up and his whole body squirms, as if he knows in advance that he's going to have fun with this child. He likes adults well enough but he doesn't show the same enthusiasm for them.

So the child playmate seems more joyous, more fun. And the baby, being by nature a fun-lover, identifies with the older child. He feels, "We are the children, the happy-go-lucky children—in contrast to our serious parents." If there is a third or fourth child in a family, they tend to have the same personality traits and attitudes as the second. The first-born has had no child companions to play with or to identify with. He is simply the third person in the family. He assumes he is in the same category as the other two—a small adult. When he is perhaps two or three years old and the second child comes along this doesn't make the first feel, "We two are the children in this family." Instead he sees that the new baby is a helpless, fretful, diaper-soiling infant, and this strongly reinforces his conviction that he is not in that category at all, that he acts and looks much more like his parents. He is not a big baby; he is a small adult. He identifies with his parents. He says condescendingly to his mother, "See, he can't do anything! He can't walk! He can't talk! He can't eat! He just makes messes." This is not the only basis for him to decide that he is more like an adult. It helps him mightily to ease his jealousy to see how much more of a capable, grown-up person he is. He doesn't need to compete with the baby as a child because he's more like a parent.

It is important for the first child to have help in overcoming his jealousy since he is subject to greater jealousy, on the average, than later children in the family. This is because he has had his parents all to himself for the first few years of his life and assumes that this is his permanent privilege. When the second comes along and the child becomes aware that the parents are giving this baby attention and love, it comes as a much greater shock and betrayal than the second feels with the arrival of the third.

You may be wondering why I am making such a point about how the second child identifies with the first child and sees himself as a child, whereas the first identifies with his parents and sees himself as a small adult. This is the main basis, I believe, why second children tend, on the average, to have different personalities and attitudes than first children. The only child has some of the same reasons to identify with his parents and adults, in general, as the first child. He doesn't have the problem though of sharp jealousy that the first endures with the arrival of the second.

The outstanding trait of most second children, it seems to me, is easy sociability. He makes friends quickly, effortlessly, enjoyably. This is in sharp contrast with a majority of first children who are somewhat shy and self-conscious in approaching strange children; they get their feelings easily hurt if a strange child is grabby, rude, or just lacking in cordiality. This is largely the result of the first child's having lived mainly with parents and other adults who have been consistently considerate, kindly, and affectionate to the child.

The second child has run into similarly rude children but has been so eager to make friends that he has ignored the impoliteness; and the strange child has been won over by his friendliness.

Second children are less likely than the first to get high grades in school. They enjoy life too much to worry about grades. Grades are parents' concerns, at least in the beginning. Second children are less likely than first children to go into the "helping professions" such as teaching, medicine, social work, or nursing, in which the professional acts like a parent in helping out the younger or less-fortunate individuals. Second children are more likely to get into business where enjoyment of competition is one of the major motivations.

Second children are much less likely to become bossy. First children get that way because they identify with their parents, and because they try to lessen their feelings of rivalry by denying that they are children at all. On the average, second children are less serious and less responsible than first children.

The second child's rivalry with first child usually takes the form of constantly trying to catch up or preferably, to do better than the first. If the first throws rocks into the lake the second tries to throw more or farther. The second is apt to feel that the first gets more of the parents' love, though this may not be true at all. The rivalry of the first child more often takes the form of being mean, belittling, taunting. However the second can be mean to the third. On the surface, you usually see most clearly the second child's rivalry with the first, a rivalry tinged with hostility. But underneath there is apt to be a great admiration for the prowess of the bigger, stronger, and smarter first child.

I've heard a number of parents say that they found it easier to get along with their second child than with their first. They thought this was strange because, they said, they felt as if they understood and were more naturally sympathetic to the first. My explanation for this is that, from his birth, the parents have been intimately tied to and identified with the first. They want him to have all the capabilities and qualities that they have plus all the capabilities they don't have but wish they had. With the second and third child, they are more ready to let them be themselves .

Are there special problems in being second? I think it is quite common for the second child to feel frustrated not only by the realization that he can never catch up—in size, in stage of development—with the first, but also by the feeling, which may or may not be the truth, that the first is the parents' favorite. It's easy for the second to come to such a conclusion because the parents will naturally grant more privileges to the oldest.

The best way for the parent to counteract this kind of frustration is to realize that every child (like every adult) needs to feel that he is especially loved for his individual characteristics. The parents can compliment him occasionally on some physical or temperamental or social trait that they appreciate. Don't compare one child with the other, though. They might take him occasionally on a special treat or shopping spree. Or a parent can get a little bit mushy and say, not too seriously, "You're my baby, aren't you?"

I've known a few second children who felt squeezed after a third child was born. They felt that they could never catch up with the first, and that the pleasures of being the youngest were stolen from them by the third. If the parents get evidence that this is the problem, they can give him some babying from time to time. They may be able to help him by telling him, sympathetically, that they think he is feeling sad and angry because he doesn't have the fun of being the oldest or the youngest. Getting the resentment out in the open is a valuable step in lessening it. And it reassures the child to realize that his parents are aware of his unhappiness and of its cause.

We can see that there are, on the average, advantages in being the second—easy sociability, the enjoyment of competition, lack of self-consciousness. On the other hand the second is less likely to be a superior student or to get into the helping professions, if these are what the parents value highly. The world has need of people with a wide variety of traits, so it can use first children and second children! I'd advise parents to be happy with whatever valuable traits a child develops as long as he or she is happy too.

Loving One Child Less

"I feel guilty that I love one of my children, David, less than the other two. He's nine years old and the oldest. He irritates me almost constantly. I find myself often scolding and nagging him. In a way I feel I understand him the best and I suspect he understands me. Perhaps that's why we rub each other the wrong way. I keep resolving to be more patient and I really want to be, but as soon as I set eyes on him I find something to criticize. Sometimes he openly accuses me of not loving him and that makes me feel terrible. He bothers my husband too, but not as much as he bothers me."

The first thing I want to say is that I don't believe, from the evidence in her letter, that this mother loves her first child less than she loves the others. There are different feelings and actions that go to make up parental love and I am quite sure that this mother has them in ample amounts. I suspect that she would make the same sacrifices for him as for the other children. She'd go into a burning building to rescue him. She would care for him endlessly and devotedly if he developed a serious chronic illness. If in adolescence or adulthood, he got into serious trouble, she'd never turn her back on him.

What is it then that gets a parent off on a wrong foot with one particular child? Often it is an unconscious connection that goes back to the parent's own childhood. The present child may remind the parent, at the unconscious level, of a younger brother who seemed to be the favored child, or of a father who is remembered to have been insensitive and unfair. Or the mother may have felt totally unready for the pregnancy with this child. Associations like these may make the parent impatient with one child right from infancy. The child may then react with a lack of a strong attachment toward the mother, with a lack of cooperation, with a slight peskiness, which the parent sees as inborn traits of the child and as full justification for the parent's irritability.

So it's likely to be these small causes of parental impatience based on unconscious associations going back to the parent's childhood—nothing as dramatic or important as insufficient love—that makes one child less comfortable to deal with. The parent's slight irritability sets the child's teeth on edge, making him a little less cooperative, less pleasant than the average to deal with. This gives a further boost to the parent's intolerance, which is now close enough to the surface to make the parent feel guilty, since the parent suspects it is due to lack of love. The guilt is apt, in turn, to get the parent to try to overlook the child's next misbehavior or perhaps the next after that. Sooner or later the parent's attempted patience breaks down with a show of anger. This outburst gives the parent a greater sense of guilt.

So life with this child becomes a succession of irritable episodes and scoldings. The child behaves better for a few hours after a deserved scolding but the parent's guilt encourages the child to test the limits again.

The difference with a more stable parent-child relationship is that the parent doesn't start with an unconscious irritability; the child, enjoying the warmth of the relationship, can afford to be cooperative and charming, and can pay attention to the rules most of the time. So the parent doesn't have to get angry or feel guilty nearly as often.

How can a parent break out of an irritable relationship? A first step is to relieve some of the guilt by realizing that the problem is not due to lack of love.

A second approach, after there has been a quarrel or blowup and after things have quieted down, is for the parent to have an honest, person-to-person chat with the child—not a parental scolding. It might have some of the following ideas in it: "I feel bad after I've been angry with you. I love you a lot and I want to get along better with you. But I get mad at you very easily, as you know. Perhaps it's because we're so much alike. Another reason is that when I was a child I used to get angry at my brother because I thought he was my parents' favorite. You look a lot like him and perhaps I get mad at you for that reason."

It should improve the relationship for him to know that you are concerned, love him, and want things to go better. Repeat the talk with variations from time to time. Admit your own faults but go light on his. The idea is to make him feel friendlier, more cooperative with you, not to put him in his place.

A third approach is to try to figure out how your relationship got off kilter in the beginning. Incidentally, none of these approaches rules out the others.

If you can't figure it out—alone or in frank discussions with your spouse, or with an understanding friend—it should be helpful to have regular consultations with a professional counselor. It often turns out that you come to understand your own problems not so much from the insights of the counselor as from hearing yourself explain your problems to a sympathetic listener.

Preparing Children for a Good Marriage

"They fell in love, were married, and lived happily ever after," say the fairy stories. Many young Americans assume the same outcome when they fall in love and blithely enter matrimony. Yet in America one marriage in two ends up in divorce, the highest rates in the world. What goes wrong here?

There are a few hints in the statistics. The younger

the age of the newlyweds, the less likely the marriage will last. The high school students who can hardly wait for graduation in their eagerness to be the first in the class to marry are obviously not old enough or mature enough to know what their long-term needs in a mate will be. In fact at this stage of still rapid emotional and social change, most of them hardly know themselves from one day to the next, or what they have to offer to a mate, if anything. The exciting elements of a love relationship—the sexual hunger, the sexual gratification, and the dizzying feeling of infatuation—are the dominant elements in most individuals at this age. They are in love with love. A few months later it may turn out that the qualities they thought they saw in their beloved were really their own illusions. And the less attractive qualities that they had concealed from each other or simply didn't let themselves see in the other, come to the surface.

The qualities that make for permanence in a love relationship—generosity, sensitivity to the feelings and needs of the other, a sharing of interests, dedication to common aims, whether it's to build up their savings or to have children—tend to come a little later in the growing-up process.

There are, to me, two good signs in today's otherwise gloomy picture. Many young people are now waiting until their later twenties or even early thirties to marry. And many who believe they are in love are living together in their twenties, to see whether the relationship grows stronger or weaker with time. (I'm not implying that such an arrangement will be acceptable to all youths—or their parents—and I'm not advocating living together in adolescence.)

Another statistic says that farm couples tend to stick together better than city dwellers. I suspect that a factor here is that the farm couple works hard all day, all year, in a common cause and close together even though their activities may be different. Most city husbands and wives go their individual ways all day, whether both have outside jobs or one stays home, so their occupational aims differ.

My own impression is that a majority of American children grow up from earliest childhood with the feeling that they are entitled to all the good things of life and without serious obligations—a flood of toys at Christmas and birthdays; trikes and bikes and motorbikes at the appropriate ages; generous allowances; cars at sixteen if the parents can afford them; or well-paying jobs after school if they have to earn their own cars. We take all these for granted, but they are way beyond what youths in other countries expect. More importantly, youths in many other countries are brought up with a strong conviction that they will owe a lot throughout their life to their extended family (as in Greece, for example) or to their nation (as in Israel) or to their religion (as we've seen in Iran).

To one degree or another our children expect a thoroughly satisfying marriage as a birthright, as I've observed, myself, in the attitudes of high school students. If it proves disappointing, they think they have been given a bad deal. I doubt that it occurs to most of them that a good marriage is not a gift but a relationship that must be worked on—in the beginning and all through life. It has to be cultivated continually like a garden.

I believe that as parents we have to start, almost from infancy, to give our children the feeling that they are in this world not just for their own fulfillment, though that is a good aim as far as it goes, but to be thoughtful of others and to work cooperatively with them to meet the needs of the family and the outside world. This may not sound to you like preparation for marriage. But the essence of a good marriage—or any other intimate relationship—is a sensitive awareness of the feelings and needs of others, and a readiness to respond.

A child of two years can be restrained from being mean to the new baby or to a playmate or to a pet, not by scolding but by the parent demonstrating how to pat or stroke or hug or kiss instead ("Nice baby, he loves you."). Three-, four-, and five-year-olds can be entrusted with household jobs such as table-setting and dish-drying and then complimented generously on their helpfulness. Throughout childhood, I'd try to substitute plans for the usual greedy preoccupation with what children want for themselves for Christmas and birthdays with thoughtful gift giving and the making of greeting cards. Toys no longer being used can be repaired and donated to charities.

During the school years, it's good for children to hear their parents discuss the possible solutions to local, national, and world problems. Even better is when parents serve on boards and committees for neighborhood services. Or they can participate in groups that focus on the improvement of the availability and quality of health care for all citizens (we're way behind European countries and Canada), grossly inadequate day-care facilities, many poor schools, many families living in poverty, all in the richest country the world has ever known.

I feel that when their children begin to talk about the dates of their friends and themselves, parents can make casual and realistic comments on how hard it is at first to find the right person, how easy it is to fool yourself, how many marriages break up (with great suffering to the couple and their children), how good marriages don't occur by luck or magic but by the couple waiting until they have had plenty of time and opportunities to know each other under different circumstances, and how, after marriage, each partner has to keep trying to understand and please the other.

My own inclination would be to discuss with teenagers some of their unasked questions about chastity and sexual activity. I'd agree that the sexual impulse and curiosity about sex are intense during the teen years. But at the same time, there is also a reluctance to go far in sexual experimentation, and a wish to wait until marriage for intercourse, especially in those young people raised in families with high ideals. Some of this inhibited sexual drive gets sublimated (redirected) into such fields as writing and reading literature and poetry, creativity in the other arts and appreciation of them, efforts to bring peace and justice to the world. In fact, some of the most creative people in history were quite shy sexually during adolescence. (The classical example is Dante who was inspired to write some of the world's greatest poetry by having seen but never known Beatrice.) Yet at a slightly later stage of youth and early adulthood, these reserved youths are able to express and enjoy their sexuality to the full. Therefore, reserved young people shouldn't worry about their normality or be persuaded by the taunts of their bolder friends. They should wait until they feel ready, at every stage of sexual maturation. In this way they may have more to give to their marriages and to their careers.

It's natural for a mother to be excited about her daughter's early dates and popularity. But the effect of this may be to encourage the child to overcome her inhibitions prematurely and to compete for boys and dates before she knows what love is.

What can you do if you feel that your child is rushing into marriage too soon or with the wrong person? One thing you can't do is get any self-respecting adolescent to admit that she or he is making a mistake. Furthermore, the couple can always elope. I think the best you can do is ask them as a favor to you to postpone the marriage, at least until they have known each other well for a year or more. Meanwhile I'd advise strongly against putting down the loved one. I remember obstinately sticking with a girl for two more years when I was a youth just because my mother doubted her suitability. I would try to lean in the direction of seeming favorable to the beloved, ask her or him to the house often—or better still, on camping trips or tours. There is nothing as good as roughing it to show up a person's laziness, selfishness, or incompetence!

More influential than talking to adolescents about the qualities needed for a good marriage is for parents to demonstrate them in action. Almost all parents quarrel sometimes and that is nothing to be ashamed of. But there is a big difference between insulting and sneering at one's spouse and showing respect in spite of disagreement.

However, quarrels are not the main issue. When you and your spouse were in love and planning marriage, you were trying to please each other most of the time, by listening to each other attentively, looking for agreement in opinions, finding things to compliment in each other, smiling, speaking tenderly, showing physical affection in small gestures often. Once married, there's an unconscious inclination in many cases to lapse into a ho-hum, impersonal manner. Parents should keep in mind that their children are sopping up the parents' attitudes toward each other and laying down patterns for their future adult relationships and marriages, as early as three years old.

To be more specific, little boys are setting their ideals of how they should behave in their future marriages—as well as in all other future activities—by molding themselves as much like their admired fathers as possible. They are forming their ideals of the desirable woman by loving and watching their mothers. Girls are carefully observing their mothers, to learn about their future roles as a woman, a wife, and a mother—and laying plans to marry men like their fathers. It's scary to realize what a powerful influence we parents have.

Keeping alive the pleasing, romantic, respecting attitudes is not only good for the children's future marriages but for the parents' present one.

Can One Parent Be as Good as Two?

How do you succeed as a single parent? It's an important question these days because there are more and more such families. The largest number, of course, are headed by women who have been divorced or deserted or widowed. But in recent years some judges have been willing to award custody to suitable fathers. Then there are a relatively small but growing number of women who choose to raise a child—their own or adopted—without a partner.

We can get clues about the best ways for single parents to raise their children if we think first of what children in two parent families get from their fathers and mothers.

Children in general want a mother and a father. Partly because they started out from infancy that way and developed a deep emotional dependence on both parents. It is seen in how some children beg divorced parents to get together again. Children also crave what other children have, whether it's a computer, a new style of doll, or two parents.

Back in the days when there were orphanages for

neglected and abandoned children, you could see how children who had never known their parents still yearned for them. They would create them out of their imaginations and out of aspects of the various adults they did see and liked—such as staff people and visiting parents of other children. Such children would describe for you every detail of their imagined parents' appearance; tell you how they visited frequently, what fine presents they brought, how they would soon remove their children from the institution to their fine home.

Boys and girls in families with two parents learn to think, feel, and behave like males and females by identifying primarily with their parent of the same sex, particularly in the three- to six-year-old period. A boy will take on his father's way of talking and being attracted to his father's interests. When he is playing "house" with his sister, he pretends to be the father and solemnly acts out his father's roles in the home and in the workplace. He is learning to be a man, a responsible worker, a husband, and a father himself.

If you look beneath the surface, you can see that a boy is also identifying in certain respects with his mother. I'm sure that I got into pediatrics by partly identifying with my mother's love of babies. I happily gave bottles to my younger sisters and brother and changed their diapers. It has also been said, wisely, that a boy's partial identification with his mother is how, to a certain extent, he comes to understand the feelings of girls and women, including his future wife.

A second and crucial way in which a small boy relates

to his mother is by developing a strong "romantic" attachment to her. He may declare at three or four years old that he is going to marry her when he grows up! He is too young and innocent to see the inappropriateness of this idea. But she is the one with whom he has had, since birth, an intense dependent relationship. So it is natural that when he begins to have romantic and sexual interests at around three years old—for example, playing at being fathers and mothers and having babies—he will turn to the person of the opposite sex he knows best and loves best. His mother becomes his feminine ideal; her physical and emotional characteristics will have some influence on the kind of woman he will fall in love with and marry. And the relationship between his father and mother will influence his marriage relationship, too.

Girls pattern themselves by identifying primarily with their mothers—as women, as wives, as mothers, and as job-holders outside the home. But girls also need a loving, nurturing father as much as boys do. For girls will build certain qualities into their own characters by identifying in certain respects with their father. It may create, for instance, a determination to enter her father's occupation, despite all obstacles. In a more general way, girls acquire some of their intuition about the opposite sex and how to get along with the opposite sex by identification with their fathers. (Otherwise they might find males even more strange and difficult than they do in reality now!) Also important for the development of future healthy relationships with men—not only as lovers, but as friends and fellow workers—is the "romantic" attachment that little girls normally develop with their fathers, especially in the age period between three and six years.

So boys and girls in two-parent families make use of fathers and mothers to set crucial ideals that will guide them all their lives.

Up to now I've been talking as though children get their patterns and inspiration only from identification with or attachments to their own two parents. Parents are certainly most important in intact families (and in divorced families when visitation phone calls occur regularly), especially in the formative preschool years. But in all families, as children develop and learn about the world outside the family and start to want to be independent of their parents, they come under the influence of teachers, group leaders, heroes. They form attachments to them and identify with them, too.

When one parent is remote or out of contact altogether, children will instinctively turn to substitutes—a grandparent, uncle, aunt, cousin, friend of the family, teacher, or coach, who is friendly and responsive—to satisfy their need for the absent parent. It's impossible for a child to identify with someone who is indifferent to them. I can still remember the four-year-old daughter of a colleague who had been away from his family for two years while serving on the staff of a military hospital during World War II; she physically flung herself on me and took possession of me as I entered her home during a pediatrics house call.

There is no doubt—and many biographies attest to

this—that children in single parent families can grow up to be well-adjusted, successful people, because they can make do with live-apart or substitute parents. What are some of the factors that make for success or lack of it in this situation? (I'll assume, for convenience in writing, that the children live mainly with their mother, though a small minority of divorced fathers are now granted custody and in these cases the mother has the visitation rights. What I say about one parent, applies to both.)

We can first discuss the situation when divorced fathers are within visiting distance and are happy to carry out their responsibilities to their children. Children can get a great deal from a live-apart father particularly when they can visit him regularly, or if he keeps contact by other means—letters, gifts on special occasions, and telephone calls. The most effective and relatively easy way for the mother to ensure that her children get the benefits of having a father is by encouraging these visits and contacts.

The best arrangement in one sense is when the parents share custody and responsibility, and the children regularly spend a lot of time in both homes. Then the father doesn't feel so alienated. But joint custody requires a very cooperative attitude shared by both parents. Next best is frequent regular visitation with the mother having custody. But too often this ends up with the father gradually neglecting his visiting rights and other contacts with his children because he feels that he no longer has an ongoing, loving relationship with them. The mother never asks or takes his advice about child care, education, camp, etc., and the children no longer ask his opinion or permission. They don't treat him like a father and this robs him of the sense of being one. He feels that the mother takes advantage of visits to scold him and punish him (by restricting his visits) for such misdemeanors as coming late for the children or being late in returning them, for letting them eat junk food or stay up late and thereby catch colds, or for not keeping up with the child-support payments.

So an important responsibility of the mother is to foster the contacts by trying to ignore the father's faults, trying to be cordial or at least polite when he appears at her home, asking for his opinion or advice occasionally (e.g. about camp or medical or dental care), to be nice to him because it is so important to maintain his interest in the children for their sake.

If there is no contact at all between a boy and his father and no memory, he is dependent on what his mother tells him of his father and on her attitude toward men in general. If she speaks about the father's good qualities and of his love for his son and if she shows respect in general toward most men, the boy will be able to make a positive identification with this image of his father. But if she always refers to her ex-husband as a louse, this will give the boy a poor model to identify with, since he might think of himself as half louse. And if she is bitter and scornful of all men—in her talk and in her behavior—she will give a disparaging image about men to her daughter as well as to her son. She may raise a daughter who is suspicious and cold toward men. Or she may raise a daughter who is fascinated with men but who links their attractiveness with unreliability; she is drawn unconsciously toward those who have wide streaks of meanness or unfaithfulness or incompetence in their makeup, or whatever else her mother has focused on.

But many divorced women will cry out, "He was a cruel person!" or a deceitful philanderer, or an incompetent provider. This may express her feelings accurately but is aside from the point of trying to keep a good image in the children's minds—for their sake. To present the right picture to the children the mother can, with a great effort, think and speak about the qualities that made her fall in love in the first place and of how the father loved and was proud of the children in happier times.

The less contact a boy or girl have with their father, the more valuable it is that they have contacts with other friendly, responsive men. Those who appear indifferent are no help. A grandfather, uncle, older cousin, male teacher, camp counselor, scout master, athletic coach, Sunday-school teacher, clergyman, storekeeper, tradesman, or older boy in the neighborhood may become a satisfactory, even inspiring father figure, as biographies of successful people show. In a similar way a woman relative, family friend, teacher, or athletic coach may serve as a mother figure to a boy or girl.

Can a mother create a relationship between her son or daughter and a substitute father figure? I'd say that she can set up possibilities, but she can't make them click—that will depend on subtle matters of taste and personality that can't be controlled. If she sees that her child has responded to a relative, teacher, or acquaintance, she can tell that person what a hit he has made, and add that it pleases her especially because the child badly misses his absent father. If the person seems pleased but doesn't follow up, she can invite him to a meal—with his family if he has a family. Perhaps she can be more direct with a relative. Such steps should stimulate a teacher, group leader, or neighbor to at least show small acts of friendliness which may mean a lot to the child. For example, in my own youth and adulthood, I've always owned a blue suit with a chalk stripe through an early identification with a kind teacher and coach who always wore one. A mother can also suggest to her child enrollment in the scouts, a gym class, a swimming class, or a Little League team, particularly if she has heard that the leader is unusually well liked. She can also send the child to a summer camp.

What about a man a mother has dates with? Of course such a man may become vitally important if marriage occurs. But that may be a long way off. Meanwhile there are several cautions. Most children go on hoping for years that their mother and father will get back together again some day. So when their mother (or father) appears to be entering an intimate relation, many children have feelings of something like unfaithfulness. This is a reason for the parent to go slow as far as what the children see and hear. Sooner or later they should know that their mother has dinner engagements with men friends. But she can wait to invite a man to a meal at home with the children until she finds a person she can be proud to introduce to them. She can avoid even casual displays of affection until the children have gotten to know him and given indications of liking him. She shouldn't ask him to spend the night or reveal that she has spent the night out until after many months of increasing closeness, in which the children have participated.

What I have said about a mother not showing evidence of too quick intimacy applies equally to a father. It's sensible to give this advice to both parents because it's a common reaction to the pains and humiliations and name-calling of a divorce for both parties to flaunt their affairs, as if to prove that they are attractive, despite their lack of success with each other.

If the mother is falling seriously in love and thinking of marriage, she should listen to what her children say about the man, tell them she's considering marriage and that she wants to hear their opinions. This does not mean that she should give them veto power over a marriage. Many children who enjoy the company of their mother's man friend may turn suspicious, jealous, and hostile when they realize that this person may be planning to become their stepfather. In fact, it may take them several years to accept him as such. It's wise for the couple before and after the marriage to encourage the children to express their feelings toward their parent and toward the stepparent.

Several single mothers have phrased an anxious

question to me in the same words: "How can I be a good father as well as a good mother, especially to my boy?" I think there are three misunderstandings here. One is that a mother has to be a father in the sense, for instance, of teaching a boy how to throw a football or of talking to an adolescent about sex from a man's point of view. Another misunderstanding is that a boy has to learn such matters from a parent. The third is that women and men know entirely different things about life and are ignorant about the opposite sex. A mother doesn't need to become an athletic coach to her son. He can learn more comfortably from school coaches and other boys. She knows enough about sex from the male as well as the female viewpoint to talk to her son and answer his questions. Many mothers do a better job talking with their sons about sex than fathers do, since a majority of men are notoriously shy and evasive at this job.

I've explained earlier that men and women are not ignorant of each other's thoughts and feelings. There is a considerable amount of intuitive cross-knowledge between the sexes, more in some individuals, less in others, learned by identification with the parent of the opposite sex in early childhood. So mothers should not worry about trying to be fathers to their sons. They have other important contributions to make.

A mother should not remarry primarily to provide a father for her children; that should be incidental. She should remarry only if she loves the man deeply and is as confident as she can be that he'd make a good husband. The same is true for fathers. Then, sooner or later, the new parent will probably be accepted as a good stepfather or stepmother.

The Pains of a Stepparent

Years ago, I wrote an article about the problems of stepparents which I thought had a lot of wisdom in it. But when I became a stepfather to an eleven-year-old girl, I found that I didn't know beans about actually being one. Frustrated and unhappy, I went to a counselor who specialized in such matters. She gave me relief and hope by saying that I had been living in a fool's paradise if I thought I could be accepted by a stepchild in a year or two. So I didn't have to accept personally the entire blame for my failure. I settled down to work on the problem, with the help of regular family therapy, and the insights I gained from reading the increasing number of books and articles on this increasingly common problem. With divorce doubling in the past fifteen years, it's not surprising that more of us have become stepparents.

I'll start by boldly declaring that the step-relationship is just naturally accursed, just naturally poisonous. It's no accident that the villains in so many fairy tales and novels are wicked stepmothers or cruel stepfathers. They seem that way to the children involved, whatever their true characteristics are. For a stepparent is someone who barges in between a child and parent whom she has had to herself in an unusually close relationship since a divorce or the death of the other parent. The child didn't fall in love with this outsider or give the interloper permission to take up half or more of the true parent's attention. So the stepparent stirs up fierce feelings of jealousy and resentment. To justify these, the children must exaggerate the stepparent's defects and ignore the good qualities.

I'm focusing on the negatives of course. Young children do sometimes beg their parent to remarry and may be quite cordial to the stepparent. But underneath the surface, the readiness to turn bitter is usually lurking.

The children's resentment shows up as unfriendliness, uncooperativeness, and rudeness. These sooner or later get under the skin of the stepparent, even if she or he is really an unusually understanding, patient sort of person. The stepparent eventually gets cross, disapproving, perhaps openly angry. The children, who are ready to believe the worst, see this as proof of hostility. It justifies them in behaving worse.

The stepparent reproaches the parent for having brought up such badly behaved children and keeps asking that they be corrected. So the children see the stepparent as trying to turn their parent against them. The unhappy parent feels torn. To make a move in either direction will hurt and alienate someone.

In my own experience as a stepparent, Ginger had her mother pretty much to herself—in the sense of having no serious competitor—from the age of seven when her parents were divorced until I came on the scene when she was eleven years old. Mary and I fell in love on our first meeting at a conference in California, where she was then living, so we were partly committed before Ginger had even had a chance to meet me. She was robbed from the start of any feeling of participating in the choice.

Next, Mary and I, in our enthusiasm for each other, gave too little weight to Ginger's feelings. Mary came to the Virgin Islands for a visit, so that we could get to know each other better, and also to see if she'd like living on a sailboat. Since my retirement as a medical school professor, I lived on a sailboat every winter in the Virgin Islands and every summer in Maine. Ginger was left with good friends during Mary's first two visits to the Virgin Islands, but she was reported as being unhappy and uncooperative. So on the third trip we invited her and a friend. Ginger was cool to me and rude enough on one occasion to make me explode with anger.

As Ginger grew older and bolder she was able to reproach us specifically for making her feel unloved, neglected, and abandoned. We were certainly guilty of ignorance and insensitivity, but I don't think it was all as one-sided as Ginger's feelings told her.

When we planned to get married, ten months after we met, Ginger pleaded that we make our residence in Arkansas—where she had grown up, where she was the adored first grandchild on both sides of the family, and where her father lived. We agreed to settle in Arkansas; Ginger and her father agreed that she would live with him during the months of the year when we might be sailing. But when the house was finished a year later, he changed his mind, wanting her all the year or not at all. She lived with us in Arkansas spring and fall, sailed with us in the Virgin Islands at Christmas and spring vacations. She adamantly refused at first to accompany us to Maine which she pictured as friendless and always cold. When, a year later, she finally consented to go, she had a great time on shore with a dance company and with friends, but declined to sail with us unless we applied unpleasant pressure.

We took her to an international children's camp and festival in the Soviet Union, where I was invited to observe child care. Another summer we took her to Salzburg, Venice, Paris, and Tokyo, where I was speaking. At other times when Mary and I were sailing, Ginger stayed with friends in Arkansas, but it was never an ideal solution.

One summer, in response to her plea, we stayed in Arkansas for July instead of Maine, but she spent almost all her time "uptown" instead of inviting friends to our place by the lake as we urged. We saw very little of her and regretted our decision to stay there.

It seemed to me that for the first three or four years Ginger rarely looked at me or spoke to me. When she came home from school, she'd rush through the living room to her room without a word or a glance in my direction. I'd say "Hello" but could hear no reply. When I mentioned this, she answered "I said 'hello' but too quietly for you to hear." When I'd drive her to school because she'd missed the bus, I'd try to make conversation but got nowhere except for a muttered yes or no. Once or twice a year, I'd explode, "Ginger, in my seventy-five years I've been acquainted with thousands of people but none of them has been as rude as you." I thought I saw a faint smile of triumph.

As if I didn't have enough trouble just being accepted, I compounded my problem by showing my criticalness of Ginger and by trying to correct her. She picked her fried chicken into small pieces with her fingers and let her fingers dabble in the gravy. (Mary was sure she did this to taunt me.) She absolutely refused to wear her tooth-straightening headgear and I tried to make her. What madness! She kept her room in utter chaos and every morning left her washcloth in a soaking wet ball on her washstand—no matter how many times I explained that it couldn't possibly dry that way and would get mildewed.

The more frustrated I became, the more I seemed compelled to criticize her—for example, for not being considerate enough about visiting friends (according to my adult New England standards), or for saying, "Me and him were late for school."

Ginger and Mary had to live very frugally, but after our marriage, Ginger always ordered the steak or lobster at a restaurant. She quickly spent her ample allowance for clothes each month, at the best shops, and then begged for loans. I felt I was being played for a sucker but when I protested, she asked coolly whether it wasn't true that I earned plenty.

She told us stories about the lavish generosity of her friends' fathers in regard to their daughters' clothes and cars. Her implication that we should be at least as generous, and ignoring the advantages that we did provide never failed to make me angry.

Because Ginger was doing less and less well as a sophomore in high school and would never have been able to get into a university with admissions standards, we sent her to boarding school against her wishes. She couldn't imagine being happy there. Actually she was unusually popular with girls and boys at the new school and did much better academically. But she took the position, as her father did, that we were only sending her there to get rid of her, despite the fact that her father had gone to boarding school and enjoyed it, and that I testified that boarding school was the happiest period of my adolescence.

I felt that in all these arguments Ginger came out the victor since I never could persuade her of the reasonableness of any of my positions and, in fact, my attempts only seemed to convince her further about my meanness.

I often wanted Mary to reprimand Ginger, but naturally she was reluctant to do anything that would make Ginger feel she was siding with me against her. Mary told friends that she felt her arms were being pulled out of their sockets by Ginger and me. It did comfort me a great deal when Mary listened sympathetically to my complaints.

Eventually Ginger and I became good friends most of the time. How did we get that way? The first factor was time—three or four years of painful relations, then four or five years of very gradual improvement. But also Ginger was moving from an age when she was still dependent on her mother toward an increasing desire for independence. So I became less of a threat. I think that we also came to understand each other's fears and to realize that we would survive our own.

It has helped that I sometimes side with her when she and Mary argue. She now occasionally refers to me as her dad, which warms my heart—not that I want to displace her father. But when we occasionally get into a discussion of some problem of our past relationship, her recollection and mine are still so different that you would think we were talking about two entirely different families.

In retrospect, I believe that we could have become friendlier somewhat sooner if I had had the sense and the self-control to avoid criticizing her. All the experts who have written about the step-relationship agree that the stepparent should go slow in trying to become the disciplinarian. It only makes the child say or think, "You are not my parent and I don't have to do what you say!" But that doesn't mean that a stepparent has to accept abuse, only that he or she should wait for a lot of acceptance before trying to take over the kind of responsibility and guidance that is a parent's responsibility.

Should I have given up sailing for a few years? It would have been a severe deprivation and I'm not sure it would have made a difference in our basic relationship. If it didn't, I would have been doubly resentful.

Counseling could have been helpful for Ginger, but

she grimly refused to go, except on a couple of occasions after which she maintained that she had no need—meaning that the fault was Mary's and mine.

There are many more problems in stepfamilies than the one I have focused on. In some cases both husband and wife in a new marriage have brought their children into a family, and the two groups of children have to get along with each other as well as with their respective stepparents. There are the relationships with the ex-spouses, often full of continuing bitterness over visitation rights and money matters. There are the various reactions of children of different ages and different temperaments. Helpful books that deal with these and other difficulties are:

How to Win as a Stepfamily, by Emily and John Visher, Brunner/Mazel Books, New York, 1991.
The Step-parents' Survival Guide, by Hilary Boyd, Sterling Publications, London, 1998.

Are Grandparents Important?

Parents, are, of course, the most important relatives for children. This shows up dramatically for example when young children express their fears about loss of a parent—during real events such as a natural disaster or at the time of imaginary thinking. They say, "Who will take care of me if my parents die?"

But do grandparents have something special to offer? I think they do. In the first place, sensing that they are utterly dependent on adults for their physical and emotional security, children value any and all relatives as backups for their parents. I've heard them counting their kin when talking with friends: "I have two grandmothers—and our grandfather and five uncles and five aunts and nine cousins." I think that children sense that a grandparent has more security value than an uncle or aunt because the latter usually have children of their own who have first claim on them.

Of course, grandparents are as variable as people of other ages—perhaps more so—and have different degrees of popularity with children. Some grandparents have become quite intolerant of the messes and noise that children make. I had two grandmothers like that, about sixty years old. They wore black lace dresses with high lace collars held up with whale bone strips. Their facial expressions suggested disapproval. We grandchildren were taught to be absolutely quiet and polite in their presence as if they would otherwise fall apart. There aren't many now who look as fragile as they did, though there are plenty still who get tired and irritable when they are with children for more than an hour or two.

There are other grandparents who enjoy children more than they ever did when they were young parents. Many of them have asked me, "Why couldn't I have had as good a time with my own children when they were young?" I believe the main reason is that parents are endowed by nature with a great sense of responsibility about their children's health, safety, good behavior, and good character. They feel compelled to keep saying things like "Put on your coat, it's cold out," "Careful, crossing the street," "Say thank you to Mrs. Jenkins," and "You must always tell me the truth."

When you're a grandparent you can take a parent's pride and pleasure in a child's good qualities yet not have to feel responsible for every act and trait. Furthermore, as a grandparent you can be with the children as long as you are having a good time and then, when you've had enough or find them irritating, you can usually turn them back to their parents!

I well remember, when my children were young and I would have to go away for a couple of days on a professional trip, how I missed them, thought of their delightful qualities and asked myself, impatiently, why I had to keep criticizing them so much of the time when I was with them. I'd make a firm resolve to lay off the nagging and show more approval when I was at home. But as soon as I got there, I felt the old compulsion to watch and correct, watch and correct. I don't mean that I was scolding all the time, but I didn't show appreciation and pleasure enough during the times when I was with them. There's no doubt that children are very sensitive to warm approval and blossom under its glow.

At the other end of the spectrum is the tendency for some grandparents to spoil children—by giving them too many gifts, treats, and privileges or letting them get away with a lot. I don't think it does any serious harm to children to be indulged occasionally by a grandparent. Children are very adaptable. They can adjust to a lenient grandparent or to a severe teacher without getting mixed up at all about how to meet the expectations of their parents. (In a similar way, they know how to get along with a mother and a father who differ somewhat in their method of discipline. It becomes a problem only when a parent allows the child to play one parent off against the other.)

Spoiling causes trouble if a grandparent lives regularly with the family and often gives the child privileges of which the parent disapproves, or contradicts a parent's instructions to a child or criticizes the parent's management of the child in front of the child. Such behavior on the grandparents' part is not simply an inclination to indulge the child, out of kindheartedness; it reflects an ongoing conflict between grandparent and parent, inappropriately focusing on the child rather than the real issues.

One of the advantages to a child of having a fond grandparent or other relative nearby is that when a parent has been disapproving or punitive in a way that seems unfair, the child can get comfort by going to the grandparent, who only has to say, "Granny knows how sad you feel sometimes, and she loves you very much." The grandparent doesn't need to undercut the parent; that would be too interfering. She doesn't need to reinforce the parent's discipline. She only has to show sympathy.

It's one thing when a grandparent is more indulgent than the parents, which is merely irritating to them. It's quite another matter when the grandparent is distinctly more severe, wants to punish the child or shows hostility in other ways. The parents would be right, I feel, in deciding that they won't tolerate a grandparent's behavior that scars or intimidates their child. Usually it's enough for them to speak firmly and with one mind telling the grandparent that this is not their method and they want it discontinued. If this doesn't succeed, they can ask the grandparent to move out or discontinue visiting. Using a more gentle approach, they can continue to make brief visits to the grandparent, not staying long enough for the grandparent to tangle with the child.

What can the parents do with a grandparent who lives in their home or nearby and interferes too much and criticizes the parents' management in front of the child? This can drive the parents crazy especially if they are young and still feel under the grandparents' control. It's important that the parents come to a unified front by discussion and then present their view to the grandparent; for sometimes the parent who is the child of the grandparent will stand up for the grandparent against the other parent, and this puts an intolerable strain on the marriage. One or preferably both parents can explain specifically what is wrong and what they want instead. This doesn't have to be done in an angry or disagreeable manner, though usually the parents have to feel angry inside to dare to talk up to a dominating grandparent. In fact, if the parents can act firm but calm, this will impress the grandparent more than excited accusations would.

I have seen in many families where the parents love

the grandparent, but they can't get him or her to come around to their way of treating the child. For example, the grandparent insists on pushing or forcing food, or wants to keep tickling the baby to the point of hysteria, or insists that the child sit close to them in a playground when the child wants to play on the apparatus, or scares the child with boogie man stories. It's true that some old dogs just can't learn new tricks. If parents see that, despite many patient explanations, they are getting nowhere, they must either put up with the grandparent's mishandling, if it doesn't seem to be too harmful to the child, or they must keep the grandparent away except for brief visits, during which they are present.

A grandmother who enjoys children is particularly important in the life of a girl or boy who is living in a home with a father but no mother because of divorce, illness, or death. Similarly a grandfather has an extra contribution to make to a boy or girl living with a single mother. An attachment to an accepting grandparent, which is valuable even to the child living with both parents, is especially crucial when one parent is missing.

If a grandparent asked my general advice I'd say: Enjoy your grandchildren to the hilt. Try not to do things in a way that's bothersome to the parents, no matter how strong your convictions. Discuss difference of opinion with the parents but admit to them that they have the final say. Don't overload the children with presents or talk. What they'll love you for best are the conversations in which you really listen to their stories and show interest in what they tell you. If you listen without disapproval, children will enjoy telling you more and more. And their stories and comments are delicious to hear.

The Interfering Grandmother

Right at the start I want to say that most grandmothers I've known are wise, tactful and helpful, just who an inexperienced mother would want for advice, assistance, and reassurance.

But there are interfering grandmothers who won't wait to be asked an opinion. She makes suggestions about every aspect of the baby's care; and all her suggestions run in the opposite direction from what the mother is actually doing. Some grandmothers don't limit themselves to suggestions. They say firmly "You should———" or "You shouldn't———"

From my early years in pediatric practice, I have a fifty year list in my memory of some of the things that grandmothers have criticized young mothers about. For example, a mother has read that many babies are overdressed (true enough) and leans in the direction of underdressing her own. Nothing worries a grandmother more than to see her grandchild skimpily dressed or covered—it drives her frantic. I remember a letter from a desperate grandmother commanding me to write to her daughter to tell her that she must put warmer snowsuits on her children in wintry weather. I could picture this mother's amazement if she got such a letter from someone who had never seen her children or their snowsuits!

At the time in the 1940s, when pediatricians shifted from absolute rigidity in infant feeding schedules to flexibility and urged mothers to let the baby decide how much or how little formula to take at each feeding, a great wave of anxiety swept over grandmothers who had been taught and practiced rigid feeding schedules. The domineering ones couldn't help but condemn the new doctrine to their daughters—it seemed like anarchy.

Here are other shifts in pediatric practice in the past forty years that have worried grandmothers and stimulated the bossy ones to harass mothers:

A *pacifier* as a comforter for fretfulness and thumb-sucking was disturbing. Pacifiers had previously been considered "filthy and disgusting," and still were so considered by many grandmothers, long after the shift.

Toilet training used to be vigorously carried out in the first and second years. Then it was realized that it was wiser to wait until the third year, when children themselves come around to it. But this seemed like neglect of health and good habits to many grandmothers.

The custom of *removing adenoids and tonsils* for such far-fetched reasons as the simple enlargement of these tissues, or for frequent colds, or for poor appetite and slow weight gain or for nightmares, was finally abandoned. But many grandmothers (including my mother) felt that this was a deplorably backward step.

I have listed some common reasons for grandmotherly anxiety, due to changing pediatric practice beliefs.

But of course there have also been hundreds of individual causes for worry and interference. One example is insignificant baby rashes about which the doctor has reassured the mother but the grandmother remains unconvinced; or noisy breathing in the first year which may be quite scary until the doctor has explained it as a benign condition, not harmful to the baby—but the grandmother still wants more consultations. The grandmother of a baby who is a little behind average in the development of physical abilities such as sitting and walking but whose mental and social development are clearly more advanced than average, may keep undermining the parents' confidence that the child is normal by repeatedly calling attention to behavior which she is convinced points to mental retardation. This one is especially hard for the parents to take.

What makes some grandmothers so determined to control the mother? First of all, it's anxiety. It's fear that this young parent doesn't know enough. It's fear that the doctor, who may well be younger than the grandmother, is insufficiently experienced to know how to diagnose and treat the condition or fear that the mother has not reported the condition correctly to the doctor.

If you could trace the grandmother's personality back to childhood, you'd probably find that she was a worrier but tried to compensate for this by being dogmatic. I'd suspect that back in early childhood when, at one and two years, she was first trying to establish herself as a separate individual, her mother, a bossy person too, instinctively attempted to block this process by dominating her, and it was an underlying anxiety in the child about not being able to develop a normal amount of independence at each stage that made her become so insistent in her opinions, beginning later in childhood or in adult life. So bossiness is fear of being dominated, which begins in early childhood and gets passed down from generation to generation.

The problem of the interfering grandmother is worsened by the fact that she may have been dominating and undermining her daughter from early childhood. So the daughter has grown up lacking confidence in her ability to make wise decisions and—even more significantly—lacking the ability to stand up to her mother. She resents this domination, swears she will resist it, but is too intimidated to succeed at this early stage of adulthood. The most she can do is grumble to her husband and to her friends and, occasionally, get so angry that she explodes in the presence of her mother. But her mother's indignation over this "rudeness" and "lack of appreciation" puts the young mother back under her control again. I remember vividly a case in which the grandmother would telephone the resentful mother at least every other day and ask, "What are you having for dinner tonight?" The mother saw the direction the conversation would take but was too afraid, after twenty-five years, to be able to ward it off. "Corned beef and cabbage" she would answer, and the grandmother, quick as a wink, would say "Good, I'll come over, tonight." And all evening she'd criticize, openly or subtly.

What the dominating kind of grandmother instinctively counts on is the submissiveness of the mother. The mother may show this only by listening sullenly while the grandmother lectures her. Or if the mother argues back, she is apt to use, not a confident manner, but a petulant tone, as if she knows that she is licked already. And if the young mother has taken more than she can bear and suddenly explodes with anger, that too shows, in an indirect way, that she feels defeated again. It may or may not quiet the grandmother for a few minutes. But she has sensed her power again.

It's a tough problem but there are a couple of possible escapes. One is for the young parents to move far away. This may be only a partial solution because the grandmother may telephone every day or so, to get a complete rundown on the baby's situation and then give directions.

More constructive is for the mother to practice standing up to the grandmother, preferably with the help of a counselor—a social worker in a family social agency, a pediatrician or family physician, a psychiatrist or psychologist, a clergyman skilled in counseling, or a wise friend.

What the mother has to practice is how to pass off or ignore the interference before she gets mad. The easiest trick for warding off interference about health matters or daily child care is to cheerfully hide behind the doctor along the following lines: "I showed the rash to Dr. Jenks and she says it's common and harmless. It's sure to go away later and it doesn't respond to any form of treatment." . . . "Dr. Jenks says there's wide variation in the amount of sleep babies seem to need and she doesn't believe in giving any medication for sleeplessness." Then if the grandmother won't drop the topic, the mother, having given her answer, can act slightly bored or absentminded and change the subject ("speaking of sleep————") In other words, she tries not to rise to the same bait another time by repeating her answer with a little more irritation or a slightly louder voice. The messages to the grandmother are: I'm satisfied with the doctor's advice. I don't need another consultation. I'm not worried about the condition, and in fact, I'm a little bored.

This approach will take a lot of practice and there will be many failures at first. But I think it's a sound one.

Another approach would be for the mother to have a frank talk with the grandmother in which she says she feels the grandmother is expressing too many doubts about the mother's management, which is hurting the relationship between them. This is the mother's baby. She has a good doctor. The parents feel they are responsible and doing a satisfactory job. The baby is doing well by all signs. The mother wishes the grandmother would keep her doubts and criticisms to herself. But to carry the criticism right back to the grandmother in this way takes more courage than the bored approach.

Now I may surprise you by saying that when you have learned to defend yourself emotionally against the domineering grandmother, you may feel inclined to let the old lady raise her doubts whenever she's anxious and answer her matter-of-factly. The point is that when you've finally overcome your sensitivity to criticism and no longer feel vulnerable to being dominated, you don't have to fear the grandmother. After all, she can't take the baby away from you. She can't attack you physically. She's not likely to report you to the authorities!

What's the father's roles in this conflict? He should be right behind or beside the mother at all times, reassuring her that she is doing a great job and that the grandmother is off base. Furthermore he should be taking an equal part in resisting the grandmother's attacks, whether he and his wife are using the slightly bored or the frank discussion approach. Even if he thinks one or two of the grandmother's criticisms are on target, he should never admit it in the presence of the grandmother, only when he's alone with his wife. For the domineering grandmother will overuse—unfairly—any support the father gives her.

If the grandmother is the father's mother, his obligation to stand by his wife is even greater, I feel. For the interfering type of grandmother is likely, even before there is a baby, to try to come between her son and his wife, feeling, hinting or saying outright that his wife is not good enough for him. So he must be on guard against his mother's effort to get him on her side.

When the children are older, there may be other problems if the grandmother feels that, because of poor parental methods, the children are ill behaved—

slow to obey, inconsiderate, destructive, or rude, for instance. The parents can and should, I think, explain to their child that grandmother is fussy about her possessions or politeness or noisiness or whatever, and that we must go along with her wishes when we are in her house—the adults as well as the children.

If, in spite of this coaching, grandma finds things to criticize, I would advise a mild apology by the parents, and then that the parents try to cut the visit short. As a parent I'd be inclined to take up privately with the grandmother her criticisms of the children if most of them seem excessive and if there seems any hope of changing the grandmother's attitude.

But if visits remain painful despite the parents' efforts with children and grandmother, visits can be kept infrequent and relatively brief.

Vacation Without the Children

There's great variation in what parents do about vacations. Millions never get a vacation, for financial reasons. Others take the children wherever they go, because there's no one to leave them with or because the parents assume that the family belongs together on vacation just as at home. So the idea of the parents taking off without the children is in a sense a luxury, enjoyed mainly by those on comfortable incomes, or when there are generous grandparents with extra funds (or the ability and willingness to care for the children while the parents are away).

I can't picture any situation in which children might profit by being left at home. I don't think, for instance, that they'd gain any important degree of independence by a week's separation. Young, dependent ones would continue to worry. Older and independent children are already able to stand such a separation. (A sleep-away summer camp for four to eight weeks, when affordable, is different. It may help a dependent child gain independence if he or she gets past the homesickness of the first week. At camp there is a whole new life, challenging the child to become a new, grown-up person.)

On the other hand, I think that a week's vacation away from the children, but preferably with her husband, can be a great boon for an overworked mother (and what mother is not overworked), provided she can arrange good substitute care. If she can't, she may worry all the time she's away. As a matter of fact, she may worry anyway—that's one of the penalties of being a devoted mother.

Strange as it may sound, I believe from my experience as a pediatrician that the time when mothers crave a vacation most is when the first baby is two or three months old. Before childbirth, they have not had the experience of being responsible for the life of a totally helpless being, one who can't explain what's wrong except by crying. And he seems to the new parent to be crying or at least fussing a good part of the time. I was reminded of what a strain it is, recently, when I went twice to visit my new twin grandchildren (a boy and a girl) and volunteered for night duty so that the parents could get some well-earned rest. Of course the problem was more noticeable with twins, but it seemed as if there were never more than a few minutes when one or the other was not whimpering or grunting or squeaking or straining. The bottles seemed to be needed in rapid succession. Actually the twins were doing well, gaining weight rapidly, and there were long periods when each one slept. What I'm talking about is the inexperienced parent's (or grandparent's) feeling of having to be on the alert all the time, even when asleep and of constantly being needed.

The experience with the twins made me recall from pediatric practice days the intensity of the need of some beginning parents to get away and the weak excuses they gave. I'm not talking about conscientious and highly principled parents, but the less responsible ones. One mother explained earnestly that she must abruptly wean her baby from the breast so that she and her husband could attend the homecoming game at the college they had attended. Another had to wean so that she could go to Chicago to get the rest of the nursery furniture because "as everyone knows, there is almost no choice in this town!"

The biggest issue of all in whether parents can go on vacation without the children is the risk of separation anxiety, under the age of three years. We can see separation anxiety most clearly between the ages of $1\frac{1}{2}$ and $2\frac{3}{4}$ years old. The mother has decided to take a full-time job or has been called out of town to care for her mother who has suddenly developed a serious illness. She leaves the child with a sitter with whom the boy is not familiar. He is well behaved during his mother's absence, whether it's for a day or two weeks. In fact he's been more subdued, "better behaved" than he ever is with his mother. He's been deeply worried by his mother's disappearance, but at this age, the anxiety shows up as docility while she's away. The real meaning is revealed only when the mother returns home. The child rushes to her and clings. If she goes into the next room he jumps up, crying, and follows her. If the sitter comes near, he rudely orders or pushes her away. When his mother tries to put him to bed in his crib that night he clings to her with a grip of steel. If she pries herself loose he may unhesitatingly vault over the side of his crib, though he has never done this before and follow her to the door. If she can get him to stay in the bed, he may sit up, half-dozing, all night long. It can last for weeks or months.

Occasionally, as a result of an illness, a separation may last a long time. When a child stays in the hospital for weeks because of a serious acute illness, or in the case of a child with a chronic illness, and the parents visit only weekly, the child will punish a parent by pretending not to recognize her during the visits.

The treatment of separation anxiety is painful for the mother or father. The parent must avoid separations for a number of months if at all possible and must sit beside the child's crib in the dark until he is fast asleep; and this may take a couple of hours a night at first.

Prevention is better than cure. If the family can afford it, I think it's wise to hire a regular sitter or a relative, a couple of times a month, from infancy, while the parents go out to a movie or to a restaurant or to visit friends, so that the child knows from the beginning that others besides the parent can take good care of him and that parents always come back home.

If the mother knows she is going to work or go on a vacation, and the child has not had a regular sitter, she can hire one full time for at least a couple of weeks in advance of the separation, to overlap the parent. At first, the sitter just has to be there, then, gradually, do more and more for the child. When the child accepts her, the mother can disappear, first for an hour, then for longer periods.

Separation anxiety is apt to be much less if there is an older child in the family or if the father is at home when the mother is away.

Before the age of about one-and-a-half years, a child's reaction to unexpected separation from his mother may not appear as dramatic anxiety but something like depression: He looks sad, cries more than usual, and has a poor appetite. But just because this reaction may be less difficult to manage does not mean that it is less traumatic to the child's security.

Before the age of four or five months, babies do not appear to distinguish so sharply between regular care givers (mother, father, regular sitter) and other people who give a bottle or change a diaper. With very careful studies of infants, we can detect subtle differences in responses to different people even at this young age. But we know less about the effect of separation under five months. We can't say it is harmless.

Above the age of three years, children are much more easily reassured by words and they have more time sense. When a mother explains that in a few days she will be going with daddy for a rest at the beach, and when, after she is gone, grandmother or the sitter explains that mommy and daddy will be back in three more days, these words will make a definite picture in the child's mind. And he will ask questions to cover gaps in his picture and to get answers to his particular anxieties. Even at three years and older, children need to be left with a familiar sitter whom they like.

This is not to say that children beyond three years are not bothered when their parents go away. I still remember my mild uneasiness and sadness when my mother accompanied my grandmother to North Carolina for a few weeks when I was seven. But I was certainly able to understand and to cope.

I think you can guess how I would advise a parent asking about taking a vacation while leaving the child or children at home. If the child were three years or older, I'd encourage the parents to go unless there was a special problem. I'd suggest preparing the child for a week or two, so that he can ask questions.

Between the ages of three months and three years I'd warn about the risk of separation anxiety especially if there is not an older child, a familiar sitter who has frequently cared for the child, or a father who can care for the child. If the parents wish to take the risk anyway, I'd strongly urge a sitter to live-in for at least two weeks before the parents leave, gradually taking over as the child accepts her and as the mother goes out for longer periods.

Before the age of three months, when babies don't seem to distinguish sharply between familiar and unfamiliar care givers, and when some mothers feel a strong need to get away for a few days, I would encourage them to go, especially if there has been a regular substitute care giver. But if there is no regular sitter or relative, I'd suggest an overlapping period of a few days before the mother leaves.

One compromise, during the vulnerable three months to three years periods, would be to take the baby or small child along on the vacation, but for many mothers this would hardly qualify as a vacation at all. Even if sitters were available at the vacation location, the time would be too short to accustom a small child to one, especially since the child would be made somewhat insecure by the new place. It might work well enough to bring along a familiar sitter or familiar grandparent but that is getting expensive. If father and mother are so eager for this vacation at a favorite spot that they are willing to have the child or children with them all the time or to take turns, this is all right; but it's a different topic than "vacation without the children."

Trying to Keep the Holidays Relaxed

Holidays are generally fun for the whole family, not only the pleasures of the day itself, but the anticipation for days in advance and the remembrances of special events, amusing episodes, surprises, and fine presents.

But my experience as a child, a parent, a grandparent, and a pediatrician has been that holidays can easily generate a lot of stress, especially in children under six years of age and especially in the case of gift-giving holidays such as Christmas and Chanukah that whip up children's excitement and greediness. The tensions may become so intense on the holiday that, sooner or later, the young child is nervously exhausted and lets go with a tantrum.

I'll be referring rather arbitrarily to the ages at which young children are particularly susceptible to holiday tensions. Obviously, children vary a lot in their maturity at every age, so these figures are only rough average guides. Parents know their individual children's sensitivities and they shouldn't take my figures too literally.

In making suggestions for keeping holidays less tense, I don't want to sound bossy or too arbitrary. You may want to shoot the works, and take a chance on over-fatigue. However, as a parent you shouldn't feel stingy and guilty if you do want to put some limits on the amount of excitement and on the number of gifts on holidays and birthdays. After all, a very young child doesn't know what treats you decided to leave out or postpone.

Let's start with the problem of too many new experiences, at Christmas time for example. Many parents are so generous that they can't bear to leave out any treat that's connected with the holiday—the Nutcracker ballet, Handel's *Messiah,* a Nativity play, and carol singing. It's true that if you ask children whether they'd like to view any performance, they'll enthusiastically say yes. But there are several stumbling blocks, especially for children under five years old. They may get confused and tired by being engulfed in crowds much bigger than they are used to.

Young children have short attention spans and usually get bored with long performances like a concert or a full ballet. I remember taking my six-year-old granddaughter to the *Messiah* and being embarrassed when she became bored and restless and kept kicking the back of the seat of the adult who sat in front of her. I'd say that one public performance every other day is plenty. And if there is a question whether a child is old enough to take it in stride, it's better to postpone it for another year.

Then there's the question of anxiety. I'm thinking of some cartoons of Disney and Warner Brothers that may seem appropriate to parents because they are considered children's stories; but they may scare the bejeebers out of two-, three-, and four-year-old children. I heard one of the Rockefeller brothers say that after the long run of *Snow White and the Seven Dwarfs* at Rockefeller

Center Music Hall in New York long ago, they had to replace the upholstery of all the thousands of seats because they had been wet so much! There is scary stuff for young children in *The Nutcracker*, for instance.

Thanksgiving reminds one of the tensions that characteristically crop up with family gatherings. If the grandparents on both sides live within driving distance, both sets will want visits and may get hurt feelings if they are unexpectedly left out. One solution, when the children are young, is to plan with the grandparents to visit the mother's parents for one Thanksgiving and the father's the next year. Christmas can be the opposite.

If the grandparents are fussy about manners—and many are very critical—I strongly recommend explaining this to the children before the visit, coaching them about polite greetings, saying only favorable things about the food, not jumping or climbing on the furniture, playing only with objects that the grandparents indicate are to be played with, saying good-bye and thank you at the time of departure.

Thanksgiving also reminds me of episodes that can upset children in any large gatherings of family or friends. A young child may not be familiar with most of the people and may not be socially mature enough to deal with strangers who tease or question him. A friend of mine told me a story that was both amusing and sad. It was about a large family gathering, a Thanksgiving dinner at which a five-year-old boy won the ceremony of breaking the turkey's wishbone. All thirty-five family members demanded in a jovial spirit to know what he had wished for. He was obviously embarrassed to say, which made the crowd more insistent. Close to tears but convinced that he had to be honest, he confessed in a low voice, "I wanted to see Aunt Linda naked." The roar of laughter made him even more embarrassed and unhappy. In this kind of situation, the parents are entitled to interrupt with a good-natured excuse if they detect how embarrassed a child is becoming over a social episode.

I'd like to include birthdays because they are gift-giving occasions and the birthday child is the center of attention from dawn 'til the end of the party. I'd like to suggest holding down the number of guests; one handy rule is to invite only as many as the child's age. One, two, three, or four guests may not seem like much of a party to the parents, but it's plenty for a young child.

The prospect of a blizzard of gifts on holidays and on birthdays adds not only another potential source of tension, since children are intensely possessive, but it also stimulates plain greed. I can still picture my siblings and me, then my children and finally my grandchildren, on Christmases, thirty years apart, each sitting by a mountain of packages, eyes gleaming, barely able to be restrained in order to take turns. They tear off the beautiful wrappings, examine briefly each gift without any interest in who it's from, then on to the next. Inevitably one child, usually the oldest, finishes his pile first. He complains that he has no more to open. It's an unattractive spectacle of greed. And yet, this is supposed to be a celebration of the birth of Christ, who taught us about sacrifice and love.

I believe that our country and the world are in a bad way in part because of excessive selfishness. One of the main causes is that too many children are being brought up with not enough emphasis on spiritual values, particularly kindness, generosity and love. Religious holidays give us wide open opportunities to teach these values instead of greed.

I feel that the parents should make sure that presents are opened one at a time, that each child who is able to print names should keep a list of who each gift is from, and write a thank-you letter, if only of one sentence. I suggest that the whole family attend a service on religious holidays. It's worth it to keep the meaning of the holiday in focus. I'd even suggest it for agnostic families if they don't feel that this would be too insincere.

To remind children that giving is as blessed as receiving, parents can emphasize homemade gifts that children can make for relatives and friends, such as painted or crayoned pictures, necklaces made of glass beads, model planes that come in all degrees of complexity, or homemade greeting cards. Children love to make things and to give presents they've made. They only need to be reminded.

3

Contemporary Culture

Changes in the Care of Children and Old People

With a life that spanned the entire twentieth century, Dr. Spock witnessed many cultural changes that each had an impact on raising children. He was also interested in the condition of old people and the effects of cultural, political and economic change on the quality of their lives.

At ninety years of age, I've seen a lot of changes—in the care of children and in the care of old people. I despise euphemisms such as golden-age, retired people, senior citizens.

When I was a baby we didn't get solid food until a year of age. We boys didn't get a haircut until we were two or three years. Mothers hated and postponed this sign that babyhood was over, and it was fathers who had to insist. We boys wore petticoats and dresses until that age too. There were no washing machines or diaper services, so mothers had to wash all the diapers by hand and hang them on the line. And for the rest of childhood, all the masses of cotton clothes (no drip-dry fabrics in those days) had to be similarly washed by hand, dried, and then ironed (no electric irons, either) and brought up out of the basement in huge creaking basketfuls.

Kitchen stoves were fired with coal or wood and whoever did the cooking had to be an expert in keeping the fire going. There were no quick-cooking cereals. The oatmeal or wheat cereal had to be started the evening before, and kept simmering all night in a double boiler. There were no cans or jars of baby foods; they had to be cooked and then strained. You had to mix, sterilize, and bottle the formula yourself.

There were no vaccines—except against smallpox— and no "wonder drugs." The only treatment for pneumonia, ear abscesses, scarlet fever, and other infections was to pray and "force fluids."

The main differences in the situation of old people was that they did not have Social Security, Medicare, and Medicaid. So they had no financial help from the government, only the funds and securities that they had managed to save or had inherited. A majority then, as now, had not been able to put aside any substantial savings, except perhaps for a house which they were extremely reluctant to part with.

So a majority were dependent on their grown children or had to go to the "poor house."

Now, Social Security, Medicare, and Medicaid provide substantial help for a majority of retired people.

However, there is a sizable minority who are not covered. And there are many more old people who are still alive. A lot of the employed relatives, to whom older people without insurance might turn, have suffered a loss of income in the past dozen years or so, and they can't easily make the required sacrifices.

I have seen, in my own case, how old people are more subject to many diseases and have more trouble overcoming them. For example, I have experienced these conditions with old age: bronchitis, skin conditions, urgency about getting to the bathroom, a pacemaker to counteract my heart irregularity of long standing, and a "blood thinner" to keep me from having another stroke.

I am thankful for having had excellent medical care all along and for having Medicare and Social Security to pay my doctors for their services. I have also had the benefit of a second wife in my older years who is full of energy and a devoted caretaker. She doesn't let me neglect our twice daily meditation, our stretching exercises, our daily swim in the YMCA pool in summer in Camden, Maine (the ocean is much too cold) and in the ocean in the Virgin Islands in winter. For a year we've been on a macrobiotic diet—grains, beans, vegetables; no meat, chicken, or dairy—that is credited with warding off arteriosclerosis (blocked arteries), cancer, infections, and other conditions. I also give credit for my longevity to my mother's family, a majority of whom lived until their late eighties or early nineties.

There is a phrase, the "sandwich generation." It refers to the fact that many young couples are taking care of their children and taking care of their own parents at the same time.

To be sure, there are more grandparents these days who, because of insurance, can pay their own bills if these are kept modest. But that fact doesn't negate another fact: that many old people need emotional and managerial support. It's especially true in the case of a widowed grandmother who formerly left most of the decisions and the management of their affairs to her husband now deceased. It's also true of the widower grandfather who is of the dreamy, absentminded type and whose very practical wife always took care of all the details of their existence and steered him around. It's in such cases, as well as in cases where both grandparents on one side or the other are alive but having trouble keeping track of things and making decisions, that it can make hard work for the sandwich generation. It's most often the mother of the children who shoulders the job of being a mother for the grandparents. She shouldn't make all the sacrifices but should draw her husband into the decision-making and plans of action, especially if the old people are his parents.

One aspect of aging that amazes me is how different grandmothers are nowadays from what they were when I was a child.

How did grandmothers change into women who today look and act the same as younger women, in clothing, in driving their own cars, in moving briskly; perhaps in taking an interest in politics, finances, or athletics, in taking their own grandchildren on excursions or horsing around with them at home? It's wonderful!

Can You Raise Children to Make Their Own Decisions?

More and more children, I think, are growing up with a diminished ability to make their own decisions, to get involved in their own projects and hobbies, to make their own plans, for the weekend or for the next summer. They sometimes say, "There's nothing to do around here" or "What shall I do?" In other words they are more passive than they could be. And this disposition, once it's well established, is likely to persist.

There are a number of possible causes that may operate separately or together. One that I blame particularly is too much television watching (the average amount of time for television watching among American children is twenty-one hours each week!) which turns the energy and resourcefulness that are normal for children into a state of hypnotized paralysis. This is because the programs are so full of unnaturally exciting happenings. I'd say that a half hour or an hour of television per afternoon or evening is plenty.

Another factor that squelches decision-making is when parents overschedule their children with after-school lessons, from ballet to music, so that there is simply no time left for a child to dream or think up original games, alone or with friends. Another cause, I believe—and some teachers and parents will scold me for saying this—is too much homework, which leaves too little time for the child's own interests. There are exceptions such as science projects or library research that the child chooses and carries out independently, which provides valuable training in initiative and responsibility. A study made many years ago showed that homework, in the way of more examples of the same sort that were done during school hours, does not lead to greater comprehension or higher grades. Yet some teachers just load it on, in the belief that it's valuable, or at least that it impresses the children with the importance of the subject. The answer here is for parents who are opposed to too much homework to make their opinions known at P.T.A. meetings and perhaps in a discussion with the principal.

More important than homework is the philosophy of the school system and individual teachers. Do they foster initiative, responsibility, and creativity by giving the children opportunities to practice these virtues at every turn in the day's work; or do they only teach conformity and passivity by telling the children what to think, what to do, at every step? Here again the answer is vigorous discussion of the aims of education, and of this school in particular, at P.T.A. meetings. It also means electing to the school board candidates who stand for high enough salaries to attract first-rate teachers.

A situation that discourages initiative and decisiveness is when an extraordinarily close relationship develops between a young child, let's say it's a boy, and his mother that is overly dependent and overly demanding on his part. He expects a lot from her, partly because she has always lavished a lot of attention on him. And he is quick to complain to her or blame her whenever life is at all disappointing. Partly this is because she always seems ready to accept some of the blame, a bit submissively, even though she's not the least at fault. She may not be even slightly submissive, to her other children. In some subtle way or other she seems to feel guilty toward this child, ready to let him scold or punish her.

I've been describing a mother-son relationship but it could just as easily have been mother-daughter, father-son, or father-daughter. Is it possible to raise children so that they aren't likely to be complainers, or overly dependent in any other way, so that they readily take the initiative, make their own decisions, and carry them out? I think it can be done, with a little practice.

The first step is for parents to realize that children just naturally develop initiative and demand independence as they grow. By six months old, they want to hold their own bottles. By a year they want to hold the spoon to feed themselves and they want to climb stairs. By two years, they determinedly copy many of their parents' actions. By five years, they want to learn about letters and numbers and words. By midadolescence, they are fascinated with the opposite sex, whether they are shy or bold in showing it. The point is that parents don't have to push these interests, they spring from the inside. When children are allowed to follow their own initiatives, they not only develop particular skills as they come due; more important, they learn to trust their ability to take on future initiatives of other kinds that haven't presented themselves yet. They become bolder, more independent, more self-motivated in spirit.

The parents' cue is to recognize that these are valuable qualities for a successful life of any kind, and to stand back and let them develop.

I'll list some of the ways in which inexperienced or overprotective parents may interfere, unnecessarily. They may hover anxiously, especially with a first baby, instantly taking him down when he tries to climb on a low stool, on the couch, or on the stairs. It's amazing to see how cautious most babies are when testing new skills, how rarely they miscalculate. Of course, you can't let an infant crawl upstairs when there are no banisters. But I would let him run the risk of rolling off a piece of low furniture onto the floor. I'd resist the impulse to jump up and stand near, or to keep warning him to be careful.

If you have to take away a dangerously sharp or breakable object, don't emphasis the "no! no!" aspect of the maneuvers but quickly offer a safe object in its place. Of course, you have to introduce prohibitions, one or two at a time. You have to stop a baby from yanking the cords of table lamps and from chewing on the wires. You may have to remove the baby or the object a few times, saying "no! no!" at the same time. But to keep from having to forbid too many objects at first, you can get most of them out of reach ("baby proofing the room").

Give playthings that you don't have to be warning against using—blocks, cartons, wheel toys, dolls and stuffed animals, rings that fit on posts. Let the baby or small child make harmless mistakes and correct them himself.

Some beginning parents don't block too many actions but they discourage initiative by pushing objects on the child, suggesting actions that the child hasn't thought of yet, taking over and complicating some game that the child has started, because the adult sees a new angle.

When a baby or child has learned a new skill, whether it is simple or complicated, it's good for him—and for you—to recognize his achievement and act pleased, in a quiet way. But when parents in their eagerness to congratulate, exclaim for five minutes or act as if this was the world's most amazing triumph, it's as if they were taking over the child's accomplishment, in their pride. It's the child's satisfaction that's most important. And some children get such an appetite for praise from being praised too much that they are constantly demanding that their parents watch and congratulate them long after the achievement is old stuff ("Daddy, watch how I jump in the water! Daddy, Daddy, watch how I do it again!").

As children get into elementary school, they have different drives. Back between three and six years old, they were strongly oriented toward the family, boys striving to be like their fathers in manners and interests, being devoted to their mothers, thinking a lot about someday being fathers themselves, wanting to play "house," which is family. Girls are focused on their mothers; they aim to grow up to be just like them, and think of having babies as the most exciting aspect of life.

But by ages six and seven, subconscious rivalry with their fathers steers boys away from playing "house" and husband and father. They turn, with relief and pleasure to impersonal abstractions such as reading, writing, arithmetic, science, and nature. That's why in industrial nations academic schooling begins at six years, because children are ready. Girls go through a similar shift.

Instead of trying to be as much like their fathers as possible, boys want now to imitate their peers, in messiness of clothes, in crudeness of speech and table manners (elbows on table, noisy guzzling of soup, absent-minded kicking of the table legs). To conscientious parents it seems that all their careful training is going down the drain, and they tend to nag. But it's really a forward step in that children are sensing that they must gradually outgrow their parents as models and try to fit into the big world beyond the family.

It's wise for parents at this age to try to limit their scolding and restrictions to important issues and to ignore the minor ones like table manners and washing hands before meals. I'd say it's an age when parents should try particularly hard to allow their children to take initiatives and make decisions—about projects, about hobbies (it's a great age for projects and hobbies), about how to organize their possessions, and their rooms (even if it looks more like disorganization), about how to spend afternoons and weekends, about who are to be their friends. The point is that though children's habits are apt to be irritating to the parents at this age, they are rarely harmful—to the child or to the parents' possessions. So this age period offers a six-year stretch in which children can practice and strengthen their initiative and decision-making abilities, before the much more troublesome period of adolescence begins, when differences of opinions are likely to bring children and parents into more stressful conflict, and when teenagers' determination to do things their way may get them into real difficulties.

But suppose that your nine-year-old had already grown up somewhat dependent on you, and that on a vacation morning he complains that there is nothing to do around here. I would try, on the one hand, not to go patiently through the motions of suggesting a dozen activities. He could think of them himself if he was in the mood. What he's really trying to do is make you feel responsible for his being out of sorts, and he'll scornfully knock down any suggestions you make. On the other hand if you just show your impatience with him, he'll nag you some more and you'll both get more irritated.

I'd try to surprise him and snap him out of this stale and fruitless game by walking over to him, taking him by the shoulders, and saying, "You know plenty of things you could do. But really you are only trying to make me feel that I'm the one who has to think up something new and entirely different. Well, I can't. You'll have to think it up yourself." He might try a little longer to complain but I'd walk off, cheerfully, and go about my business, as if I didn't feel any obligation at all.

Parental Guilt from Working Outside the Home

When both parents or a single mother have full-time jobs outside the home, it's common for the mother to feel guilty about not being at home with her child except in the evening. I think that the single father or a father in a two-parent family might feel the same guilt if it had not always been the tradition in our society, at least until very recently, that child care was primarily the mother's responsibility. This guilt may be felt by the parent whether the child is in a day-care center, a family type day care, or cared for in the child's own home. Parents can also feel guilty when a "latch-key child" of school age returns to an empty home or just hangs around the neighborhood after school lets out.

The most common form for this kind of guilt to take is for a mother to feel that she should be a slave to the child's wishes when she finally does come home, to make up for her absence, no matter how tired she is. She'll read him stories or play checkers for hours if he demands it. She'll serve his favorite foods night after night even though she is thoroughly bored with them herself. I've known a few mothers who brought home a gift every day and the child always asked, "What did you bring me today."

A more subtle symptom of guilt is when a mother or father puts up with chronic disagreeableness, rudeness, whining, or lack of cooperation in a child, which an unguilty parent would not tolerate for long.

We hear a lot these days about "quality time," meaning the enrichment, the strengthening of the relationship between parent and child when they are together, rather than satisfaction with simply being in the same house or the same room, without much communication.

In one sense there is a conflict between my advice to parents not to feel obligated to be a slave to a child just because you have only limited time to spend together, and the contrary sounding advice I'm giving now about how to make the time together close, personal, highly satisfying to the child. I'll try to clarify my ideas about the difference.

Certainly it's important for parents to realize that their children value and deeply enjoy their time with their parents, especially when they sense that there is a personal, special appreciation of each of them as an individual. To turn this around, we hear bitter complaints from those who felt that they had very little time with their parents while growing up, because the parents totally absorbed themselves in a career or in social affairs.

A crucial difference to the child is whether the attention flows freely from the parents or has to be badgered out of them by the child's demands and complaints.

Certainly parents resent giving the attention that a child extracts from them by making them feel guilty; and they can't correct that resentment altogether. The parents' reluctance to give the attention can make some children even more demanding of attention or at least more grouchy about the lack of it; so a sour cycle is set up and maintained.

But the attention that comes spontaneously and unexpectedly from a parent, because the parent is freely loving and thoughtful, has a sweet taste to the child, and even a little of it has a good effect—an invitation to have lunch at a restaurant, a shopping spree, a visit to a museum, attendance at a sporting event or movie.

One of the ways a mother or father can avoid resentment about being constantly asked to give too much attention is to be cheerfully frank with their child about which hobbies, games, or books the parent enjoys and which ones bore her; then they can bargain. (I loved the Babar books and was happy to read them again and again. But I was not only bored, I was irritated by the deliberate illogic of some of the books that delighted my sons.)

Though I am heartily in favor of parents and children spending time with each other enjoyably, I want to express an opinion that may sound contradictory: I don't think that the amount of time together or the closeness of the communication is the only, or even the most important, measure of the quality of the relationship. The idea of parents setting aside time to play with their children, to amuse them, is a relatively new one and a particularly American one. In the traditional, developing parts of the world, children are watching their parents attentively, identifying with them, copying their every move during play from about two to eight years old. Then gradually they take on a sort of apprentice role in real-life activities, boys going fishing with their fishermen fathers, for instance, a girl taking over from her mother the job of carrying the baby of the family on her hip. In these traditional societies, the parents don't "play" with their children. The children first play at being parents. And then, as the children grow older, they gradually take on roles as genuine assistants to the parents.

This is not too different from America as recently as the early part of the twentieth century. My father didn't deliberately play with me. But he was hospitable to me and explained what he was doing when I watched him mend a shelf or make a crate or change a fuse or start a fire in the furnace. I don't remember our mother playing with us either. I think of her as assigning us household jobs and then reminding us to perform them.

It's not healthy for child or parent when a child becomes a chronic demander or complainer as a result of success in bullying his reluctant parent into giving him privileges or possessions beyond what's sensible. A confirmed demander-complainer is an irritating, unpopular person for everyone to deal with. He will be limited in all his relationships and endeavors by this demanding side of his personality unless he learns through many painful experiences to change his stripes.

It's not pleasant to be a parent of a demanding, complaining child. Every day the child will raise a dozen issues, small or large, with which to go after the parent. When the parent reveals guilt by being hesitant or by attempting to bargain, a child instantly detects that he has a chance of success and redoubles his arguments and pleas. This can go on and on. It exhausts the parents, making the parents irritable.

What then is the sensible way for parents to avoid guilt and hesitancy, as a result of taking a job outside the home and leaving a child in someone else's care?

I'll mention first the value of counseling. A parent might start by talking to the child's pediatrician or family physician. If more help is needed, a referral to a family social agency, a behavioral pediatrician, a psychologist or a psychiatrist will help the parent become more aware of how guilt is interfering with management, to sort out the factors leading to the parent's sense of guilt, and to resolve the conflicts as far as possible.

As a parent becomes aware of how her guilt is interfering with her relationship with her child, making her kowtow to his demands or complaints, and put up with his impoliteness or uncooperativeness, she can begin to practice sensible limits. I don't mean that she should become disagreeable or severe. In fact, those attitudes signal to the child that she is conflicted about what she should do. What I do mean is that she should practice giving prompt, cheerful, friendly, definite responses to his requests, even if she has to give negative answers 90 percent of the time; and that she should ask for cooperation in a positive, polite way—not crossly—as if she were asking a friend and took it for granted that the child would comply.

Of course a child who has been demanding and uncooperative won't reform quickly, nor will a mother or father who has been submissive or nagging. It's helpful for the parent to start the new system with a friendly talk about how both of them have fallen into bad habits in dealing with each other, how she or he would like both of them to change, and how this will make life together more fun.

When the child disappoints a parent, instead of complaining to him or scolding him, the parent can remind him of how they are trying to treat each other like adults and then give him a prompt, polite answer to his request, or ask in a friendly but firm tone for his cooperation. It may help both of them to be aware of the new spirit they are striving for if the mother hugs the child or holds his hand while she's speaking. This is a symbol of the new spirit between them.

The change is not easy to achieve but it can be done, and is infinitely worthwhile.

Children Speak Out About Scheduling

I had written an article for parents on how some school-age children seem to me to be overscheduled, in the sense that their parents urged them to take on so many after-school activities that they had little time for themselves or for friendships. So I decided it would be wise to ask children to speak for themselves.

We picked a private (nonparochial) school in New York City whose students come mostly from professional families. The teachers then selected ten children from the third and fourth grades who could be counted on to speak up. These children had two to five after-school activities per week, either in the school or elsewhere.

Most of their mothers as well as fathers worked long hours, not getting home until six, seven or even eight in the evening. The children in these families all agreed, with great earnestness, that they wished they had more time with parents. They didn't hold this against them, though. They accepted this as an inevitable aspect of life.

One aspect of the lives of these big-city children, whose parents work long hours, is that the parents have to provide a child-care person who would be in the apartment at least from the time the children came home until the parents arrived. No serious complaints were made about the sitters, only that most of them could not help with homework because they had not had enough schooling or they had learned by other methods.

There were several aspects of this school that I admired. One was the small classes, not more than twenty students in each class. A teacher, no matter how good, cannot pay sufficient attention to individual children, when they get perplexed, if the class is large. But small classes mean expensive budgets, whether in fees or taxes.

Another good thing about this school was a philosophy of making the work interesting and challenging rather than just demanding. Some people think that if school work is pleasant and exciting not enough is being learned. Not so. I don't mean that every class that's fun is necessarily fruitful. But children are full of curiosity and they love to learn if the work is designed to fit their capabilities, if it is presented in a challenging and interesting way, and if it is taught by a person who loves children and loves teaching them. My sons went to such schools, so I know.

A third admirable aspect of this school is that there are after-school activity groups, of considerable variety: foreign language clubs, a stamp collectors club, a computer club, a carpentry club, etc., in which the children take a lot of the initiative and there is no grading. Several children in our group spoke of participating in one or more of these because of their own interest. But they also spoke of dropping one or another because they were too busy. They clearly felt that the choices to join or to quit were up to them.

Some school administrators and some stay-at-home parents object to the idea of after-school activities in school, feeling that too much is being asked of schools by parents, and that the expense would have to be met by higher fees or taxes. I don't want to get into argu-

ments about theories of what are the separate responsibilities of families and schools. The fact is that in a
majority of families both parents now work outside the
home and somebody should take the responsibility for
supervising the children. Who is in a better position
than schools to provide space, facilities, and trained
leaders? It's a smart school administration that offers
these and smart parents who apply political pressure to
get them.

The children interviewed, just like sensible adults,
saw both sides of the issues that we talked about. At the
start of the discussion they agreed, with sighs, that they
felt too much pressure and felt tired, from activities and
long hours, on top of classes and homework. But when
questioned a second time, later, they weren't so sure,
because they liked most of their activities. They had
participated in selecting them and weren't ready to give
most of them up, though they still admitted that they
sometimes felt bored or pressured.

Several took a groaning attitude toward music lessons and especially music practice. They may have wanted the lessons in the beginning. But when they found
how slow progress was and became bored, especially by
the practice, and they wanted to quit, their parents
reminded them that the lessons would still have to be
paid for. So then the parents had to nag about practice.
I have a cautious attitude about individual music lessons and individual practice because I've heard the
same story so often, from patients and from my own relatives. Kids are sure, after hearing a musician applaud-

ed, that they could easily learn and charm audiences, despite parental efforts to instill a more realistic view. I've heard that group lessons are much more likely to retain children's enthusiasm, and I think schools should provide such group lessons. When children get to be teenagers and have more self-discipline, they may have more judgment about taking individual lessons. Of course, some children remain enthusiastic about individual lessons from a young age and are quite willing to practice, most of the time.

These children all had homework to do which added to their feeling of pressure and fatigue. I have a prejudice against homework of the usual kind, which is to do more examples of the same sort done in class or in study hall, or to answer more questions from the reader or social studies book. Many years ago an experiment showed that this kind of repetitive homework does not add anything to pupils' understanding or mastery of a subject by the end of the year. Yet many parents and teachers believe that it is somehow beneficial to children and would be upset if it were not required. I'm against it because it just keeps children's noses to the grindstone for one or two more hours, without benefit. Suppose each of us working adults had to bring home a couple of hours' worth of repetitive work each night, just because the boss thought it would be good for us! I feel entirely differently about work at home on some project connected with a school subject, such as a science project which the student selects and figures out for herself how to collect the data so that it proves some point in the end. Such projects foster initiative, independent judgment, responsibility, and creativity. I also think that independent study in the library in order to present a report to the class is valuable. It teaches children how to use the library in addition to how to take initiative and responsibility, and how to organize a paper.

I was amused that some who were single children wished for a brother or sister to keep them company in the absence of parents in the late afternoons and early evenings. But several who had brothers or sisters were able to sadly advise the others that siblings are likely to absorb the attention of parents and visitors and to interfere with your possessions and activities. Perhaps this craving for a brother or sister for company, in the apartment-house dwellers, is the same thing as the enjoyment of neighborhood friends that are available to children living in single-family houses in smaller cities or in the suburbs. In any case, none of the group we interviewed complained of not having time for friendships, though I thought there was insufficient opportunity.

They all looked forward to sleeping late on Saturdays but complained that they woke up early just as on school days. They all watched cartoons on Saturday mornings. I speculate that, although there is a violent content of most cartoons which kids of this age period seem specially to enjoy, they just love being able, for a few hours a week, not to have to do anything active—just relax and watch passively.

My final conclusions, after hearing these children, is that there is a temptation to overschedule among conscientious parents who want their children to be capable in all things. Such children do feel the pressure and they do feel tired. And to me it seemed that, compared to children of my childhood, they have insufficient time for reading (they said they read, but mostly after going to bed at night), for friendships, for home hobbies, and for loafing.

Yet they liked most of the activities they were involved in, especially those that they had clearly chosen for themselves. The boy who seemed the happiest rode the subway to Brooklyn twice a week to practice baseball with his team.

If I were a parent of school-age children today, I would carefully refrain from suggesting an activity but leave it to my children to involve themselves in those they had chosen for themselves. Then if they got themselves overscheduled, I'd let them give up any of them without reproaching them, hoping they'd learn something from the mistake.

Calling Parents by First Names

To some people, the idea of allowing or encouraging children to call their parents and other adults by first names is disturbing. They see it as an example of excessive permissiveness, in the same category as permitting children to act rude, demanding, or openly defiant. To others it is only an expression of friendliness. Some of these latter parents may explain that they don't want their children to be in awe of them or resent them, feelings that they remember harboring toward their parents at times. Others express it positively as wanting their children to think of them primarily as pals of a sort, not as authorities just because they are older.

I should explain quickly at this point that I've never advocated permissiveness though I've been accused of it by some people who've never read *Baby and Child Care.* I've always said and written that it's wise for parents to give their children firm, clear leadership and to require politeness and cooperation. But I've said, too, that firm leadership doesn't need to be at all disagreeable; preferably it should not be.

I do not think that allowing first names must necessarily be a sign of overpermissiveness; on the other hand, it sometimes is. But whether it means a simple and spontaneous impulse on the part of parents to be on a friendly basis with their children or whether it can, in some cases, have another, deeper meaning, depends on the spirit or attitude in which the parents encourage the first name manner.

When I speak of the spirit, I am thinking of whether the parents are acting simply out of loving feelings or out of the fear, conscious or unconscious, that if they behave like strict, old-fashioned parents, their children may be antagonized the way they remember being antagonized by their parents at times. This fear of alienating their children is fairly common these days. Another problem still is that so few young couples now settle down near their parents, through whom they might absorb the family's traditions about child-rearing.

I feel quite sure that calling parents by their first names doesn't by itself reduce children's respect for their parents, or make them less polite and cooperative. I've known plenty of families that prove this point. I also remember during childhood summers in fishing villages in Maine, where it was the custom for children to address all adults by their first names, being surprised and a little bit shocked to see that they got away with it. I learned gradually that it meant no disrespect and was acknowledged as acceptable manners by all adults. My own parents were old-fashioned and strict in such matters; we didn't even say Dad or Mommy, we said Father or Mother.

My older son came to the habit of first names at about four years old. We had had an unusually companionable and pleasant weekend and he began calling me Ben, the way my wife did, without any suggestion from me. I took it to be a very spontaneous, almost unconscious, way of saying, "I've been warmed by your great friendliness today." My second son, who came along eleven years later, naturally imitated the first. Both sons when interviewed as adults said they thought I had been a strict father, so my acceptance of "Ben" did not express to them a feeling that I was being overpermissive, afraid to be a firm father.

There are two quite different attitudes possible when parents allow or encourage their children to call them by first names. One is the simple, unforced impulse, of nonguilty parents, to express friendliness, lovingness. But that, doesn't mean that they think they must avoid parental leadership. Anybody who has seen families in actions, anyone who has been a child, in fact, senses that because children are inexperienced and impulsive they need parents who will guide them, clearly and firmly. But this guidance does not need to be even slightly disagreeable. It's the same for adult workers in a shop or office. They need and want a leader who makes quite clear what he wants in performance, but they want one who is friendly too.

The other attitude is the uneasy, guilty-in-anticipation feeling in certain parents who themselves were brought up with little self-confidence, because they were criticized and scolded, not necessarily to a severe degree but more than average. This left them with the fear when they became parents themselves that they might create similar antagonisms with their children. This fear of making the same mistakes makes some of them lean over backward to try to avoid the attitude of the scolding parent. Some of them try to avoid seeming like parents at all. They try to be only pals.

But though children greatly appreciate friendliness in parents, they sense that they need clear parental leadership also. They are uneasy without it. Some of them, we've learned in counseling children, misbehave with the unconscious aim of making their parents be firmer. In other words, children will have many pals, but they will have only one father and mother to be guided by. Good to be a pal—as long as you are first a parent.

When insecure parents, of the kind I've been describing, ask their children to call them by first names it may be, in some cases, in order to avoid seeming like parents. Children sense the reluctance to be parents and are made uneasy.

Parents who fear that their children will lose respect for them and turn into brats, if allowed to use first names, have put the cart before the horse, I believe. Children's respect for their parents does not depend on what words they use for them, as long as the words are not intended to be rude. Respect depends on the parents' love, fairness, dependability.

Although I have focused on the different meanings of the first names that some children call their parents by, what I've said about parents' guilt versus self-assurance and firm leadership versus wanting to be only pals really applies to all aspects of child-parent relationships. But using the example of children's first names for their parents seems to me like a clear way of presenting the underlying attitudes and the broader problem.

It would be easy enough for me to say that parents who are afraid that first names will lead to disrespect should accept my reassurance. But deeply held beliefs can't usually be given up on somebody else's say-so. Parents should only accept advice when it feels right to them. Otherwise it's apt not to work right.

People who are afraid to be firm parents find it a long, tough job to overcome a lack of self-assurance that goes back to their early childhood. In fact many of them don't even realize that they are hesitant or apologetic in the management of their children. But if they see the problem, see how uncomfortable it is for themselves, and see how it fosters a nagging attitude in the children, they will be encouraged to work on it even if results come slowly. Sympathetic counseling will help in most cases.

Teenage Idols, Punk Style, and the Early Stages of Sexual Development

Why do teenagers and preteens go in for such a bizarre appearance as the punk look? Why are they moved to tears by a rock star's performance? Why do they threaten their lives with tobacco, alcohol, drugs, and loveless sex?

For answers, we have to look at the motivations of adolescents, at peer pressure, at their unconscious search for an adult identity, and at the ambivalent stage of their sexual development in the preteen and early teen years.

At the simplest and most obvious level young teenagers are wild to grow up, as children of all ages are. But young children just want to do what they see older children and adults do, whether it's to learn to read or ride a bike. In the preteen and teen years, they want to do more grown-up things, too, but the emphasis is on wanting to appear sophisticated, to seem older and more worldly wise than they really are. This element of self-consciousness is what's so different and so strong. I remember my amazement when I happened to walk by a huge junior high school for girls in New York City at noon when hundreds of twelve- to fourteen-year-old girls came pouring out onto the sidewalk. It seemed as if every one of them reached frantically into her pocket or purse for her pack of cigarettes and lit up. Here were dozens of future cases of cancer and heart disease being started, not because of addiction yet (since their use of tobacco must have been fairly recent), not because of pleasure yet (for there was a lot of uncomfortable coughing), but simply because smoking is thought to be sophisticated-looking and, at this age, slightly wicked. Obviously the surgeon general's warning of death was feeble by comparison.

The need to appear worldly is complicated by peer pressure, which is powerful and has two sides. There are your peers who want you to join them in something that is forbidden or at least disapproved of, such as cigarettes or alcohol or drugs or sex. It makes them feel more comfortable if they can recruit you and others into these sins. Or, if they fail to persuade you, they can feel bold and courageous to have had the courage to do what others don't dare do.

The other side of peer pressure, the stronger side I think, is the adolescent's own sensitivity to pressure, the almost desperate need to conform to the standards of friends, the distress at feeling an outsider, a namby-pamby, a queer duck. The self-consciousness is painful. I remember when I was in boarding school (which I loved) and my parents made the kind effort to drive several hundred miles to be with me at Thanksgiving.

But more powerful than the pleasure of having them take me and some friends to the inn for a fine dinner was my anxiety that my friends would see that the back-seat of the car was a mess with loose possessions or that they'd notice that my mother's back hair had gotten loose from the bun and was curling down over her coat collar. A generation later my son would let us come to watch him swim in his high school meet, only if we promised to behave in a sedate manner and pretended, by not greeting him or applauding him, that we had no connection with him.

In the adolescent and youthful years (I call youth the period from about seventeen to twenty-one years old), the unconscious process of finding an adult identity plays an increasingly important role. Adolescents and youths must finally give up their identification with their parents and find their own adult selves, not simply in such obvious categories as what occupations they want to enter but, more importantly and more deeply, what kinds of people they will be, with what feelings and ideals, and with what basic relationships they will have with others.

There are several factors that determine the final outcome. First is the temperament they were born with. Second is the particular relationship each had with their parents throughout childhood. Third is the intensity of the rebellion against the parents in adolescence. And finally, what elements in the parents' makeup they will incorporate as parts of themselves as they emerge from rebelliousness and settle down in adulthood—as workers, as spouses, as parents, as neighbors and friends.

Some individuals go through a minimal stage of rebellion and soon glide into adulthood with characters and attitudes fairly similar to their parents. At the opposite extreme are those who thrash around, sometimes for years, making themselves and their parents miserable with their criticisms and uncooperativeness. They are having great difficulty finding themselves. All they can visualize is how much they don't want to be like their parents. But they are stuck in the middle of the struggle to get free. If and when they can eventually stop differing with parents, teachers, employers, they may turn into productive people.

Now we can get on to teenage idols and why some young people act a bit crazy in their adoration. Many observers of adolescents in our contemporary society agree that we keep our adolescents and youths feeling separate and immature by making them stay in school through high school, which is seventeen, eighteen, or nineteen years of age. In college-educated families, the pressure is on them to stay four or more years longer, to get an undergraduate or a graduate degree. By contrast, adolescents in many nonindustrial societies are admitted to full adulthood and responsible jobs in their teens. In colonial times in our own society some young men became ship captains by the age of twenty-one. This kind of timetable makes them feel fully grown, responsible, and respected at an early age.

In our society, many youths feel unconsciously like

children and part of a separate society. This childishness shows up, I think, in the playful riots that sometimes erupt on college campuses in the spring. In a hospital in which I was an intern, the house staff had a binge in the spring, part of which was a mayonnaise slide extending the length of a long, long corridor.

What I'm leading up to is that our adolescents and youth feel excluded from the adult society, so they retaliate by creating a youth culture of their own which accentuates the differences from the adult world. They invent their own slang, their own clothes styles and hair styles, their dances. They honor the bands, the singers, and the tunes that appeal particularly to them. And if their choices in any of these fields baffle or irritate their parents so much the better. I remember my impatience in adolescence when my mother said in disgust, about my favorite jazz tune, "How you can hear anything appealing in that kind of noise . . . I don't see it!" It was remembering my mother's words that kept me from saying the same thing about the rock music my stepdaughter adored.

There is a further element in the hysterical adoration that ten- to fifteen-year-olds, especially girls, display for the singers and other performers who have an intense sex appeal. The performers' appeal can be communicated by a generally wild and aggressive manner, by bumps and grinds, by suggestive or blatant lyrics, or by all these in combination. A dramatic example of a generation ago was Elvis Presley who reduced his young audiences to screams and tears. His appeal was so powerful that the jealous fathers of teenage girls of one city tried to get the chief of police to exclude him from performing. I think that the largest element in this kind of infatuation is the ambiguous stage of sexual development in girls in this age period, beginning with the early signs of puberty development at ten and eleven years old and continuing until about fourteen, fifteen, or sixteen years old. When I say "ambiguous stage of sexual development" I mean that these children do, and yet they don't, understand the changes taking place in their feelings and in their understanding of their sexuality. This is because they are emerging from the stage that started when they were six or seven years old, when sexual feelings were under a good deal of repression and they hadn't dared think much about it. But beginning at nine or ten or eleven or twelve years old, their sexual glands start to operate and send sexual feelings and thoughts into their awareness. So they are partly responding, still partly resisting.

When a performer is sending out messages about sex that are partly hidden or disguised, the preteen and early teen child's unconscious mind, which is more wise than her consciousness, picks up the exciting sexual message. But her consciousness, which is more proper and still feeling the repression, doesn't allow her to understand fully the explicit sexual messages. However, her conscious mind doesn't object when she is enthusiastic to the point of screams about the performance and the general attractiveness of the artist.

This capacity of preteen and early teen children to

have some sexual excitement without recognizing that it's sexual is, in some respects, similar to the capacity—in girls and boys—to have crushes on adult members of their same sex, such as teachers, star performers, sports heroes, or friends of the same age and sex. The attraction, since it is not toward members of the opposite sex, may not be recognized as sexual, at least for a while, and does not seem forbidden.

Next may come a romantic crush on an adult of the opposite sex, most typically one who is safely far away such as a movie or television star or a singer, who can be dreamed about to your heart's content, without the chance of being embarrassed by inexperience. This attachment is less hectic and more private than the hysterical response to the performance at the concert.

Finally comes falling in love with a contemporary of the opposite sex in the same town. But as you remember from your own adolescence, most of these early infatuations are quite unrealistic. The child is yearning to be in love and reads into a likely looking individual the qualities he or she wants in a beloved. But it often takes only a brief experience to show that this is not the desired person at all. So it's falling out of love and falling in again, over a period of years, the choices gradually getting more appropriate.

All the stages of sexual development I've been describing used to have to be passed through and it took a long time. With the rather drastic change in sexual mores in recent years, particularly the easing of restraints and repression, the process of sexual development has been greatly hastened for many young people. But it may still be a disturbing time—for children and for their parents. Many parents have told me that with an understanding of sexual development in adolescents, they are able to accept and guide their sons and daughters through some of the tough times.

How Open Can You Be About Sex?

In the Victorian Age, which really lasted up to World War I, sex was carefully ignored in respectable adult and parent–child conversation. A pregnant woman was said to be "in a family way" to avoid the word that referred more directly to the sexual connection. Breasts were "the bust" as if this was just a region of the body, not two milk-giving, pleasure-giving organs. The genitals were not called by their real names but by cutsie words like "Tee Tee" when speaking to children. My mother, in her middle age, told me, and several of my friends' mothers told them, that they had absolutely no information at the time of their marriage, from their mothers or friends, about what sex meant and were truly shocked. From our more psychologically sophisticated perspective, we can guess that they had little conscious awareness of sex, because of the intense inhibitions with which they were raised. But having observed dogs, peeked into forbidden books, and overheard enough conversations, they probably knew more than they admitted.

In the Victorian period, most children had no friendly explanation about sex at all. For some of them there was absolutely no discussion, just grim silence, which they interpreted as stern disapproval and which led to fears and guilt, since they were at least dimly aware of their own childhood sexuality. Many adolescents were given warnings about the immorality of sexual activity and fantasies, especially masturbation, which was believed to cause insanity, damage to the sexual organs, and abnormalities in offspring.

Though there was probably more sexual maladjustment then than now because of the fears and guilt, a considerable majority did overcome their ignorance and found pleasure. In fact, the Kinsey Report of a couple of generations ago, which analyzed sexual behavior in relation to level of schooling achieved, showed that the people with university educations, who had on the average been brought up the most strictly and who came to sexual activity later in youth or adulthood, deliberately prolonged and intensified their sexual pleasure. Perhaps the forbidden aspects of sex heightened their eventual excitement. So the inhibition of sexuality in childhood did not always interfere with sexual adjustment, provided the individual had a resilient personality able to outgrow the early prohibitions.

The revolt against this conspiracy of silence and threats came first from psychiatrists and psychologists, particularly Sigmund Freud and his followers. They realized that sex is natural and normal, meant to be enjoyed, though it is a lot more complex in humans than it is in other animals. Freud concluded, from the psychoanalysis of many patients, that sexual awareness is felt by children by the age of three and four years old. This is shown by their curiosity about genital differences, wanting to touch their own and each other's genitals (that's the appeal in playing doctor), their endless playing of "house," which means pretending to be a married couple and to care for a baby. Observations by psychologists and pediatricians since Freud have shown us that babies play with and explore their genitals even in the first year of life.

A preschool-age boy falls in love with his mother, declares he is going to marry her some day. He yearns for physical closeness and exclusive possession. He puts his mother on a pedestal as his feminine ideal; aspects of her personality and appearance will influence his choice of a wife later. At the same time, he greatly admires his father and patterns himself after him. A girl, in a similar way, falls in love with her father and tries to become just like the mother she looks up to. They are practicing to be ideal husbands and wives and parents.

At the turn of the century, many professionals who cared for children were concerned with the connections between sexual maladjustments in adults and the often weird fears and excessive guilt about sexuality that many patients showed, presumably as a result of parental warnings, misinformation, seductions, or no information at all in childhood. Out of this grew the sex education movement, with the idea that sound information and wholesome parental attitudes would prevent these problems.

There are many sensible aspects of sex education.

Children around two and three years old notice, get worried about, and ask questions about genital differences, if they have opportunities to observe them. At around three to four years old, children begin to wonder where babies come from and it usually satisfies them to explain that they grow from a seed in the mother's uterus. Later, questions occur to a child—how does the seed get in and how does the baby get out. Children are apt to assume that, like food, the seed is swallowed. Then the parent can explain how the parents' loving feelings make them want to hug, how the father's penis enters the mother's vagina, and the father's seed enters a tiny egg in the mother's uterus.

It's wise to remember that the clearest of explanations get mixed up with children's fantasies, and that their questions need more answers at each stage of development.

Beginning around six years old, it's more comfortable for children to learn about sex in animals; some schools keep a pair of guinea pigs in a first grade or kindergarten class at least for a while.

The average age for the start of puberty development in girls is ten years and in boys the average is twelve years; but variations as much as two years earlier or later are common and should be explained at home and in school. Menstruation comes, on the average, at twelve to thirteen years old. Some early developers are embarrassed, and late developers worry that they are abnormal and will never get the normal sexual changes in their body or a growth spurt. Knowledge about normal sexual development can guide parents in their discussions with their children about sex.

In addition to parents, wise teachers, not only in biology but English and history and social studies, make it easier for adolescents to bring classroom discussions around to their own feelings about such matters as the right age for makeup and dates, curfew hours, chastity, contraception, pregnancy, and marriage.

More important than the content of what you say to children is your manner in saying it. The aim is to make them feel comfortable about having asked, so that they'll feel free to ask again and again. Many parents will find this harder to do than they imagine. For most of us have been brought up with at least a little anxiety and guilt and this may make us tense up when the questions come, make us take on a lecturing tone. I don't mean that this will spoil the discussion, but that if you know the problem ahead of time, you may be better able to soften your reply.

It's easiest to deal with a two-, three-, or four-year-old's questions because these children have not yet become self-conscious or on guard about sex questions. You might say that they put their parents at ease with their own casualness.

Adolescents present special problems. They are intensely aware of sexuality in themselves and in their friends. But they don't like to think of their parents as having sexual feelings or a sexual life. ("I thought they were beyond that sort of thing," they say.) Girls may or may not bring up discussions with their mothers—it depends on their personalities and their relationship. Boys are unlikely to bring up such topics with their fathers, and most fathers are similarly inhibited. I remember vividly, with each of my sons—they were eleven years apart in age—waiting for an ideal occasion when we were in a car for a relatively long drive. I said, gingerly, "Maybe this is a good time to talk about the facts of life." Each boy said, hastily and nervously, "I know all about it already." I doubted that that was true; but it was evident that neither found it easy to talk about sex with their father. So I blundered on with a little lecture, anyway. Our way to get around this difficulty is to say to an embarrassed adolescent, "Here is a book. If you have questions, I'll be glad to discuss them." It is sometimes the mother who, because of the failure of the father, has to discuss sex with her son. It was that way with my mother.

I believe that the new, wholesome attitude toward sexuality that resulted from the sex education movement and other tolerant psychological and sociological trends has been a tremendous improvement over the anxieties and guilt induced by the Victorian policy of condemnation. But this great shift has also brought changes that I consider unfortunate. It seems that a majority of teenagers now take sexual activity to be entirely natural and harmless, their birthright. This encourages, to some degree or other, a casual attitude, promiscuity, pregnancy, and venereal disease. It's a strange phenomenon that, despite all their sophistication, a great majority of sexually active teenagers obstinately decline to use any contraceptive. When pressed, they give various reasons: They haven't become pregnant in the past, so they won't in the future. Or they don't like to admit that they will continue to be active, they prefer to think that their past sexuality was an exception resulting from passion that won't be repeated. Or some of those who feel unloved at home dream of loving a baby who will in turn love them. Some who are more angry at their parents allow themselves to become pregnant to shame them. Obstetricians, with whom I've discussed this problem, say that the only solution is for the parents to take these children to the doctor for very specific instruction in the various contraceptions. Even then, the parent must insist that the contraceptives be actually used—a message for both boys and girls.

In this day of single-parent families, it is said that an occasional mother may make an adult confidante of her daughter or son, even about intimate aspects of her life, and that this robs the child of childhood. It's natural enough for a parent without a spouse to want to turn to a responsive child for companionship and confidences. Whether it warps the child's views of life and self depends on how far the parent goes. I think it's all right for a mother, for instance, to speak of a new man acquaintance, especially one whom the child has met, mentioning his good and not-so-good traits of personality, and to ask the child's opinion. Obviously, a school-age child will have an opinion and will be glad of an opportunity to express it, before the relationship gets so intense that the mother won't want to hear anything critical. But in my view, it would be a mistake for single parents to volunteer details of their quarrels or of their sexual relationship. But if they are having a sexual affair and a child asks about it directly or indirectly, it's better to be honest.

I think it's advisable for a parent who has been recently divorced not to act too excited or demonstrative toward a new date in the presence of a child. Children below the age of about fifteen years are usually opposed to the divorce of their parents, hope against hope that they will get back together, and feel that it is unfaithfulness when a parent becomes sexually interested in another person too soon. So I believe it's wise for the parent to go slow, to arrange heavy dates elsewhere than in the home at first, and to let the child get acquainted with the parent's friend in a casual setting, at home or in a restaurant. Then watch for the child's reaction, and be guided by that. Young children may beg a mother to remarry so that they can have a father in the home; but when an actual candidate appears, the desire may change to rude antagonism, especially in the case of a boy, who is more likely to resent a male intruder and rival than a girl is.

In concluding, I'd like to express my opinion that in some respects the campaign to remove the inhibitions and the prudery about sex has gone too far. I'm thinking of the way so many movies show an explicit scene of intercourse and sometimes rape. Throughout the world and throughout human history, people have felt that intercourse is so intimate that it demands privacy. To show it and view it in a theater represents, I feel, a lack of respect for sex and, in the case of rape, an enjoyment of the brutalization of sex. I have the same feeling of discomfort when so many people are using the crude four-letter word for intercourse as an exclamation or a taunt or an adjective, in company.

I believe that the tolerant attitude toward sex that is now prevalent makes many adolescents and their parents forget that sex, in the broadest sense, is a powerful spiritual force, not just a physical one. This is what makes people fall in love, not just seek sexual satisfaction. This is what makes them idealize their mates. It's what makes them strive to build good marriages and to be sound parents. And part of this spiritual force is sublimated into love of the arts and nature, and into a drive to serve humanity and God.

So, it's important to keep the spiritual aspects of sexual love in children's awareness, to balance the anatomical and lustful aspects. In talking with preschool children about the origin of babies, parents can speak about fathers' and mothers' loving feelings for each other that make them want to "make love," and how they want to have babies to love and care for. They can remind older children and adolescents that though youths are likely to fall in love and out of love a number of times, until they learn who is right for them, they eventually do find a person who they yearn to live with and care for, and with whom they want to bring up and cherish fine children.

Even more to the point, parents should remember that it is their example which teaches and inspires their children most. So they should show tenderness and respect for each other even though they may quarrel at times. They can show their dedication to their children and their love for each other.

4

Discipline: Teaching Children Expectations for Behavior

Hesitancy in Parents

The most frequent difficulty between parents and children in America, I believe, is parental hesitancy—in giving directions and in seeing that they are carried out. I don't mean that it occurs in a majority of families but it certainly exists in a large minority. It's a problem for highly conscientious, highly sensitive parents even more than for casual parents.

To make sure at the start that you know what I'm talking about, I'll give you examples that I've seen often when I've been a guest in homes of friends.

A mother says in a surprised tone to her eight-year-old daughter who has been watching television in another corner of the living room, "Charlotte! It's nine-thirty! You should have been in bed half an hour ago!" Charlotte bristles noisily, "Why do I have to go to bed at nine o'clock? None of my friends have to go to bed that early! Last Saturday you let me stay up till then!" The mother, instead of becoming firm, looks slightly crushed by the passion of Charlotte's retort and turns back to conversation with the guests. The child turns back to the television. Half an hour later the mother exclaims in a shocked tone, "Charlotte dear! It's ten o'clock! It's a whole hour after your bedtime! Hurry upstairs right away!" The child doesn't act the least bit contrite. She's watching her mother out of the corner of her eye to detect whether she has reached the point of anger, decides she hasn't, and takes a chance on delaying a little longer.

A mother asks her four-year-old son who's playing in the backyard, "Do you want to come in for lunch?" He says, "No." She says, "You'll get too hungry." He answers, "No, I won't." She says, "I've made spaghetti." He's on a negative track now so he answers, "I don't like spaghetti," though he really loves it.

On the first snow day of December a mother says to her twelve-year-old daughter who is about to walk to school in her good, new shoes, "Wear your galoshes or rubbers." The girl answers, "Nobody wears them." The mother, thinking that this may be true and not wanting to embarrass her, drops the matter.

The common denominator in these examples, some of which may not seem important enough to you to be worth arguing about with a child, is that the parents in these stories do want their child to do something or other, but are easily put off when the child objects. This

wouldn't be important if it was only an occasional difference of opinion. But I am thinking of families in
which this is a regular pattern. The parent is usually
hesitant or slightly apologetic in making requests and
the child, counting on this indecisiveness, has developed a habit of arguing or silently ignoring requests. In
a sense the child has the parent on the defensive. The
child has gained the upper hand.

I remember this parental uncertainty when I began
pediatric practice in New York in the 1930s. But I don't
remember it when I was a child in New Haven, from
1903 to 1920. My mother never had the slightest doubt
about her opinions or her methods in child care.
Occasionally, I or one of my sisters, feeling that she had
come to an unfair judgment, would try to persuade her
to change her mind or at least to lighten her punishment. But she never budged. None of the mothers of
my childhood friends were as severe as she, but I don't
remember any of them being wishy-washy either. If I'm
right, the trend became evident in the 1920s and 1930s.
Where did it come from?

I believe that the main factor was the multiplying of
psychological theories in the first quarter of the twentieth century, the increasing numbers of psychologists
and psychiatrists, and their acceptance by so many
American parents. Their books, articles, and lectures
made it clear for the first time that children's behavior
and misbehavior were related to the way they were managed by their parents. (In earlier times, parents had
blamed the devil or heredity.)

An unfortunate and inaccurate statement that came out of the mental-health movement and caused much parental distress said, "Behind every problem child there is a problem parent." Views like these made sensitive parents feel quite guilty; they jumped to the conclusion that such common, minor disturbances as thumb-sucking, nail-biting, below-average grades in school, and fear of dogs, meant that they had seriously mishandled their children.

Another influence came from the psychiatrist, Sigmund Freud, who made profound discoveries about the mind. He was most influential in America and pointed out the presence of hostility at the unconscious level between parents and children, the harmful effects of excessive guilt and also of excessive repression, and the normality of sexual impulses even in early childhood. These observations were true, but they were unfamiliar and disturbing to most parents at first.

John Watson upset parents from another direction by insisting that any desired behavior in a child could be taught if the parent was sufficiently determined. If you wanted your child to be a musician, play music to him constantly during infancy and early childhood. He said that kissing, hugging, and comforting a child were harmful to the development of a healthy and strong character. He said that shaking hands with a child once a day was permissible! Many American parents took him seriously.

All these new psychological concepts were heaped on conscientious parents who had no good way of evaluating them in those days or deciding how far to believe and apply them. Parents felt unsure of themselves, ignorant and guilty. Many of the less confident parents came to feel that only the professionals knew how children should be raised, that parents were more likely to do wrong than right and that, when in doubt, it is better to do nothing. Another confusing aspect of this psychological revolution was that the experts often appeared to disagree with each other. One would be reported in the newspaper as saying that cruel fairy stories are harmful to young children. Another would declare that they are a healthy outlet.

Another explanation of how sensitive, conscientious parents become guilty and indecisive in our psychology-minded society, is that they feel badly about the harsh way so many children were treated in earlier times and they also feel guilty about the tensions that sometimes existed between themselves and their parents. They want to avoid such hostilities at all costs. So they lean over backward at any sign of resentment in their own children and quickly withdraw their requests or their corrections.

A factor that has made new theories about children attractive to many parents has been the disappearance of the extended family. In earlier centuries, young parents lived near or even with the grandparents and other relatives and were in frequent communication. That's how they got their advice about child care—in small, easy doses, from people they trusted and were comfortable with. Gradually they acquired their confidence and their own beliefs.

Nowadays young couples often live hundreds or thousands of miles away from their families and have to depend on the concepts put forth by the professionals they consult, or listen to on television or hear at a lecture, or read in articles and books.

Another factor contributing to parental indecision in America is our lack of long-established traditions of child-rearing. In many other parts of the world the people are of one stock, families have lived in the same place for hundreds of years, and everybody has more or less agreed about how children should be brought up.

But in America, there have been many waves of immigrants since 1620 from all parts of the world. Each group brought different ideas of child-rearing. But these people emigrated from their native lands because they were dissatisfied with some aspect or another of their lives. So America got a hodgepodge of contradictory customs from its immigrants who, in addition, were rebelling against some of them.

As a result, Americans have lacked the comfort of universally accepted beliefs. Each family has had to decide how it wants to bring up its young ones. In one sense, it is a benefit to have such freedom. But in another sense, it confronts beginning parents with tough questions, doubt, uncertainties, and, when things don't work out right, guilt.

Another factor still that has contributed to the uncertainty and submissiveness of parents is what I think of as an over-respect for formal education, the belief that you don't know anything about a subject unless you have passed a course. Certainly it's true that you don't know much about repairing a television set unless you've had quite a lot of instruction. But knowledge about child care comes predominately from the experience of having been a child, from care of younger brothers and sisters, from being a sitter, and finally from being a parent. Only a small part comes from instruction from books and people.

I've been writing as if it were only in the first quarter of this century that parents were confused, made indecisive by new psychological concepts. But the process has continued, perhaps a little less intensely, right up to the present.

A large factor in the hesitancy or firmness of parent depends in many cases on how they were treated as children. Some parents instinctively encourage their children to make up their own minds, take initiative, take responsibility and feel good about themselves and their achievements. Others lean toward cautioning their children, doubting whether they can accomplish new or difficult projects, correcting them for every mistake or fault, so that the children grow up with too little self-confidence, too little self-esteem. Either attitude will naturally carry over when their children have grown up to raise their own children.

What's the harm in parental indecision? It doesn't create delinquency or other serious behavior problems. It does tend to encourage a demanding, pesky and annoying quality in children, for they are quick to recognize and exploit ways to get what they want—as humans of all ages do. Furthermore, it is exhausting for parents to be challenged on every decision and to have to defend it or to be constantly frustrated.

Is there a way to overcome it? No easy way that I know of. In the first place, I have the impression that a majority of indecisive parents are not aware of their own indecision, though they are conscious of and bothered plenty by their children's argumentative nature. So the first step is for such parents to recognize that the irritating and exhausting peskiness of their children may be the result of their own hesitancy. If they can see this, they can then practice overcoming it, practice being firm.

I believe that many of these parents are afraid to be firm because they equate firmness with disagreeableness. They assume that if they are firm, their children will stop loving them, will resent them. But this doesn't have to follow at all. Those parents who have self-confidence, who have no doubt about what they expect of their children, who make it clear, and who don't back down, can ask for cooperation in a pleasant manner. They don't start with an irritable tone since they don't expect to be frustrated. Their pleasant manner tends to elicit agreeableness and compliance from their children.

It may be helpful for indecisive parents to know that for a parent to make the "wrong" decision is less disturbing to the child than for the child to constantly feel compelled to argue with the parent. So, in retraining themselves, parents should feel free to give prompt sensible replies to their children's requests and demands and to stick with them. When they realize that a child who kept saying, "But why can't I?" is not really asking for a reason but is only trying to wear the parents down, the parents can occasionally answer, with a laugh, "Because I know I am right" meaning that the child knows very well why, and that the parent is tired of being questioned endlessly.

Parents who are trying to break their habit of hesitancy and backing down should know from the start that it will take a long time to be fully successful and that their children will continue to badger them for many months even when the parents are partially successful in being firm. Every single time that the parent succeeds, it means a dent in the child's attitude and all the dents add up.

Now, in order to be more specific and practical, I'll go back to my three examples. I'd suggest that the mother of Charlotte keep in mind that her child now has the fixed habit of trying to postpone bedtime, and that the mother be ready to prompt her when the proper moment comes; then keep focused until Charlotte moves. If she doesn't move, even with her mother looking right at her, the mother may need for several months to take her by the hand, lead her up to bed or bath, perhaps read her a short story.

The mother of the four-year-old only asks for trouble when she asks him whether he wants to come in for lunch; this offers him an invitation to say "No." Much better to say, "Lunch is ready," or "What do you think I've made for lunch? Spaghetti!" or some other popular dish. Better still, if he's known to be balky, it would be better for his mother to go out to him, fall into conversation about what he has been doing, meanwhile take him by the hand and lead him in. If he still balks she can turn serious, say that she had cooked a good lunch and she wants him to come in now. As a last resort, I'd pick him up calmly and lug him in. He might be so angry he wouldn't eat but he would have learned that I meant it when I say I want him to come in.

If my twelve-year-old daughter told me that no one wears rubbers or galoshes even when they are wearing new shoes, I'd either say, in a matter-of-fact tone—not an overbearing one—that I want her to spare her new shoes, or perhaps offer the alternative of wearing her old shoes.

As children get into their teens you have to gradually leave more and more of the noncrucial decisions to them. But you can and should let them know how you feel about the situations that come up. And if the matter is crucial—for example, no riding in a car with a driver who has been drinking, no riding with a boy whom the parents have not met, no staying out beyond curfew unless the parents have been called and agree— the parents should be ready to give their ruling promptly without hesitation. If children want to argue, it is wise to hear them out briefly; but if you still feel the same way, say so firmly and decline to go over the same arguments again and again. By being definite and firm, you settle the argument more comfortably—not only for yourself but also for the children. For if your answer is wishy-washy, you oblige them to go on arguing.

Consistency in Discipline

Some parents think that consistency is the main element in discipline. To me, that's putting it too strongly. The child's desire to be loved by parents and to grow up to be like the loving parents, are by far the strongest factors in good behavior. If there isn't deep love in the parents there is no motivation for good behavior in the child as the childhood of many criminals show.

Another crucial factor is whether the parents respect themselves and, as a result, ask for respect from their children—no rudeness or defiance without a reprimand.

Parents should make very clear to their children just what they desire and expect in the way of behavior. Without that clarity and definite quality, children are left uncertain and they keep testing the limits, to see where the limits are. Does the parent convince the child by her manner of speaking and acting that she expects her child to cooperate and will see to it that he does?

I would put consistency next in importance. Along with the desire to love and be like parents, self-respect among parents, and making clear expectations, when you add consistency, they all fit together to make a child cooperative—not only in action but in spirit. Consistency is more a matter of rules whereas the other factors in discipline depend more on feelings; I believe that good discipline is predominantly a matter of feelings. If the feelings are good you can be relaxed about the rules. But if the feelings are sour, you can't get much success with consistency alone.

Consistency in discipline—sticking to certain rules by parents and children—makes life much easier for both. It minimizes arguments, which are a terrible waste of time, energy, and goodwill. When a child occasionally tries to break or stretch a rule, the parent who has a good relationship with her child and who means what she says only needs to mention the rule matter-of-factly, and the child recognizes that it's no use trying further. I say "matter-of-factly" because if the parent's tone is irritable or angry, the subtle message is that the parent doesn't feel entitled to have such a rule or to enforce it, which encourages the child to go on arguing.

If there are going to be rules (instead of the parent deciding each separate issue by her own personal judicial judgment), I think it is preferable for the parent to consult the child before establishing the rule. An explanation why a rule is necessary, a clear statement of the rule, and an invitation to the children to comment goes a long way to ensure success. Most children who have been managed in a fair way are reasonable about rules as long as these are not established at the height of an angry argument.

Does consistency mean that a rule can never be broken? No. Rules are a way to make parent-child relations go more smoothly; but they shouldn't be allowed to rule the family when parents and children want to suspend them. The going-to-bed hour can be modified on a special holiday or a visit from a close relative. A rule against candy, cookies, and cake can be broken when a child goes to another child's party or when the grandparents bring sweets on a visit. On the other hand, it breaks down the effectiveness of a rule if the parent allows it to be suspended several times a week. Incidentally, I think that if a parent thinks it's sensible to allow a rule to be broken, the parent should give in to the child's plea promptly, rather than make the child beg and beg for fifteen minutes and then give in. The latter encourages a child to argue endlessly on every issue, with the hope that the parent will eventually surrender.

Why is it that children are ready and willing to argue every issue or rule if given any encouragement? We tend to forget as parents that we have absolute control over our children when they are growing up and before adolescence. Imagine what it would be like if, as parents, we had to get permission from strict live-in grandparents for every action we wanted to take at home, all day long: when to get up in the morning, what to wear, what to eat, table manners at meals, how to spend our money, whether to wear a coat, what friends we could bring home, where we could go for recreation, what hour for bed. It would not be surprising if we begged, argued, whined, if we thought we could get our way. In this situation, we would accept the consistency of rules as long as they were fair, and we should have the same expectations from our children.

The Father's Role in Discipline

I once met with a group of mothers of elementary school-age children with the idea of finding a topic they'd like to discuss. We tossed around several subjects, each of which had a few supporters but none that aroused the general enthusiasm until someone suggested fathers who dodge their responsibilities as disciplinarians. Suddenly everyone in the group was eager to say her piece on this topic and, particularly, to express her resentment that her husband was one of those who shirk their duty and leave all the child management to their wives.

I remember one of the mothers sarcastically acting out the scene in her family when the three girls are meant to be in bed and quiet. Instead they can be heard upstairs giggling, chasing around, and quarreling. The mother says to her husband, "I've had to correct and nag and scold ever since they came home from school this afternoon. I'd like you to take over now. Show them that you are disappointed with their behavior and that you mean business." Then she mimes him going to the foot of the stairs and calling out sweetly, "It's bedtime, girls. Please be quiet now and go to sleep. Good night." The group of women showed their disapproval of this father's meekness and sympathy for the mother. Other members of the group gave examples of fathers unwilling to do their part.

There are several ways to understand and learn from this situation which occurs in many families. A father who has been looking forward to a pleasant evening with his wife and children hates to be cast in the role of disapproving judge and disciplinarian over episodes that occurred before he came home. He may not take the time to appreciate that his wife has worn out her patience with the children and feels she's entitled to expect the father to take an active role at this moment.

I've had other fathers say to me, "I don't want my children to resent me, the way I often resented my father." So they hope to be just a pal to their children and to avoid the disapproving aspects of parenthood, especially discipline.

The desire to be a pal to one's children can be sound, or it can be unsound. Certainly we all know parents who manage, without effort, to be friends with their children. This makes for a much more pleasant and richer family life, richer in the sense that there can be much more sharing of joys, humor, worries, much more learning from the experience of other family members. But when a father, irritated with some behavior of his son, tries to suppress or hide his disapproval because he wants to be just a pal, the son always senses the disapproval anyway. Furthermore, it makes the boy anxious when his father is trying to conceal his anger. He wonders, "Why is he hiding it?" Might it be so violent if it were released, that it would be dangerous to life? To put it the other way, irritation and anger that is expressed openly is a known quantity. It is experienced by the child and it passes. He has survived, he is a little wiser, and he feels a little braver for having gone through it.

A good father may be a pal to his son if he can also be a managerial father, who has no hesitation about providing parental guidance when it's called for.

Another way of putting this is that a boy grows spiritually to be a man by identifying with his father, borrowing strength and inspiration from him. If he senses that his father is hesitant or afraid to play the full role of father, the boy feels let down, deprived of the normal model.

I believe that a father should share equally in the responsibility for discipline of children. If a father is dodging his share, the mother may have to be the one to educate him!

A father should know that it doesn't help his son or daughter to have him go light on management and disapproval. In fact, it's likely to worry him more, as I explained. This doesn't mean that the father should encourage himself to be disagreeable or threatening or punitive. The best management, whether in a family, business, or school, is a matter-of-fact and friendly approach. It's letting the child (or subordinate or student) know where the mistake or misunderstanding lay without implying incompetence or bad intention. Then it's good parenting and leadership to make it clear what's expected, in a tone that assumes the child will of course want to do it right next time.

Most important—because it applies to all families— a father should know that when he guides his children toward certain behavior, it shouldn't be thought of as simply disapproval, or anger, as we are apt to assume from remembering our parents' faces and tones of voice when they scolded us or commanded us. The father, who is an admirable and powerful person in his children's eyes and with whom they want to identify, is revealing his beliefs, his ideal, his sources of strength, as he guides them. Much the same applies to mothers. So the children feel they gain strength and wisdom by patterning themselves after him, especially when he stays friendly and avoids cranky hostility. So discipline, in the sense of management and control, should be thought of, not as disagreeableness, but as opportunities for positive leadership and inspiration.

In some families where the father has not participated in discipline, the parents should have a serious discussion about the need to share the discipline role. A focus on the learning value of discipline for the children, when both parents participate, may help them appreciate the importance of each parent's influence on the growth and development of their children.

Lying

A four-year-old tells you that he thinks a lion lives in the bushes in a vacant lot not far from home. What does he mean by that? A five-year-old, for six months, has been reporting the doings of an imaginary playmate who frequently has fantastic adventures. Or the imaginary playmate is often blamed by your child for having done something wrong that your child actually did. Why the imaginary playmate? A ten-year-old clumsily changes the grades on her not-so-good report card. Well, here we can guess why.

There are several kinds of "untruths" before the age

of six years, and we should see the difference between them. Beginning at three years old, a child's imagination becomes known to parents and others through stories, imaginary play, and imaginary friends. This kind of imagination in preschool children can be seen as a sign of their maturing brain—both their emotional life and their thinking processes. Parents marvel at the connection between the development of imagination and language skills.

At this age children can't distinguish clearly between reality and imagination. So a four-year-old boy who loves to have adventure stories read to him and who reports to his parents that a lion lives in the vacant lot next door is not trying to deceive or gain any advantage; he is sharing a good story as his parents have shared many with him. There is no need to make a federal case out of this. In fact, a parent should see this event as a major leap in the child's development. All the parent needs to say is something like, "You made up a wonderful story."

On the other hand, a four-year-old child who often reports scary, unrealistic happenings and who shows other signs of being an unusually anxious child—afraid of other children, frequent nightmares, afraid of being separated from her parent in a shopping center—needs to be evaluated by a pediatrician or a psychologist. In this situation, the imaginary stories are a part of many other symptoms of anxiety.

If a mother has seen her three-year-old daughter, out of jealous meanness, snatch a push toy from the one-year-old boy who is crying, and the girl denies it hoping to deceive and avoid a scolding or punishment, it's a lie by any definition. It's wise, if a parent is sure from past behavior and from the guilty look, not to ask for a reason but to jump ahead to the next step and say, in this case, "Be kind to him, he loves you," or "I know you sometimes wish he wasn't here, but I can't let you hurt him." For to ask a child whether she has done wrong only invites a defensive lie and makes the parent's handling of the situation more difficult.

A young and only child has an imaginary companion with whom he regularly shares fantastic adventures. This is a common and normal event. It occurs in children with both limited and expansive friendships. However, if the child's play experiences with other children are limited, his parent might bring him, several times a week, to where other children his age play. Could he be enrolled in a nursery school or day-care center? These are ways in which, if he is starved for company, he could have his social needs met. Just as important, these are ways in which his normal need for imaginative play could be satisfied by cooperative play with other children which would keep reminding him that though the actors are real, the stories are made up.

The young boy who regularly uses an imaginary companion to blame all his own misbehavior on suggests a somewhat different problem, whether or not he is also lonely. Have his parents set such high standards that he feels constant guilt for some minor lapse or other, guilt that the average child sheds as a duck's back sheds water? If so, the answer is for the parents to ease up in their expectations.

Why not let a young child go on telling fantastic stories to his heart's content or blaming an imaginary companion for all his little sins? I certainly don't believe in squelching the creative imagination out of young children. It will be valuable all through their schooling, and in most occupations, and as a asset in social life. But I don't think we should encourage children as they grow older (beyond six or seven years old) to remain confused about what's real and what's unreal. That sometimes leads to an adult who goes through life telling preposterous lies about himself and his amazing feats, even when the lies do him no good and are sure to be exposed in time. And the adult who can never accept the blame for anything, even when his fault is evident, but must always shift the blame to others, is quite unreliable and makes everyone angry who deals with him.

It's easier to discuss lying in children of six or older, because they know the difference between truth and untruth. One of the most common areas for lying in the school-age child is schoolwork. In many schools, some children feel that they are up against rigid standards of performance. They often feel that the teacher is out to judge them, and will punish them with exposure, shame or not promote them. Parents may add their own disapproval or punishment.

There are many causes of below-average schoolwork such as below-average intelligence or a specific learning disability in reading or arithmetic neither of which may have been detected, evaluated, or led to an appropriate school placement or remediation. A child who was never read to at home or otherwise academically motivated may have limited skills for early learning. Inattention and distraction in the classroom may be the result of a temperament that predisposes a child to an attention deficit or an emotional problem that distracts attention from schoolwork.

I've listed a few problem areas to remind you of how many pitfalls there are for many school-age children and explain why there are so many temptations to lie when a child is having trouble and isn't able to explain to teachers or parents just what the problem is. The first few steps with any school problem, whether or not the child is lying, is to consult the teacher and the principal who will evaluate the problem, make recommendations about educational or psychological testing, and whether to call on the school counselor or refer to a pediatrician or psychologist.

When a child is detected altering a report card, lying about the theft of another child's trading cards, money from the mother's purse, or of an object from a store, the first step in addressing the moral issue is to have the child recognize the lie and to apologize to the person who has been the victim. The parent can accompany a bashful child or even be the spokesperson: "He is sorry; he won't do it again."

If the child has lied to a brother, sister, or friend about a broken toy, for example, the same rule about prompt apology should apply.

But suppose there is no absolute proof that the child has lied. I said earlier in regard to the young child that to ask him if he lied is likely to get you only another lie. And each further time you ask the more obstinate he becomes. It is much more effective, when you are almost certain of a lie because of past behavior and present appearance of guilt, to say, "I think you lied to me (or to someone else). I want you to always tell me the truth, and I will tell the truth to you, so that we can always believe each other." Then, don't wait for him to answer that statement, but go on with the need to apologize to the person originally lied to; if it was somebody other than you, make plans for a prompt visit. If it turns out that you were mistaken, apologize sincerely. And if you don't have enough evidence to accuse, don't make an issue of it, let it go. If he is actually beginning to experiment with lying, there will be future occasions to get the problem out in the open.

It may not seem to you that apology is enough of a punishment. But children are more deeply impressed by what parents do than by any lecture, and the picture of the parent hurrying with the culprit to confess to the victim is a vivid lesson.

Besides, in the handling of any moral problem it is better for the parents to continue to show a basic trust in the child, to act as if they assume the child will behave better as soon as he understands how people feel about the misbehavior, than if they act horrified and rejecting, which may harden his heart.

If a child, despite detection and apology, goes on

lying regularly, it shows that the problem goes deeper than if it occurs just once or occasionally. Then the need for a consultation with a mental-health clinician—a developmental-behavioral pediatrician, a psychologist, or a family social service agency—is necessary.

But whether the child's lie is the first one or whether it has become a regular pattern, it is important to show by your behavior that you still love him, want to remain close to him, and have trust that he will give up lying sooner or later.

5

The Social Development of Children

Play: The "Work of Early Childhood"

To adults, play means such games as swimming, base-ball, or golf, indulged in for pleasure alone. We sharply contrast play with work which is essential for keeping the family alive but which we usually do not consider pleasurable though it may give satisfaction. Everything that children do spontaneously, we condescendingly call play, implying that they are just amusing themselves but not carrying out any serious purpose. In making such distinctions about children, we adults show that we are confused by our own attitudes toward our own play and our work.

Most of children's play is very intense work, designed and dictated by their emerging instincts to bring about learning and maturing in vital aspects of development. But at the same time children's play is exciting and pleasurable—that's what lures them into it and keeps them working at it until they are satisfied that they've mastered that stage of it.

An eighteen-month-old boy reaches into a wooden box and removes a dozen colorful blocks. He carefully places them in a row on the floor or struggles to stack several on top of each other. Then, one by one, he tosses the blocks back into the box only to haul them out a moment later for a new round of arranging and stacking. He repeats these steps over and over again, studiously absorbed with this activity until he is called for dinner.

A two-and-a-half-year-old girl clutches a purple crayon and scribbles vigorously on a sheet of paper. Although she seems riveted by her work, she makes no effort to depict an object or person. She simply goes through the motions of drawing, moving the crayon this way and that, pressing as hard as she can on the paper.

An adult onlooker might conclude that these children are enjoying some simple fun and games. Yet for very small children, drawing a picture or building a block tower requires just as much concentration and effort as learning later to read or adding columns of numbers. When they are finished, they might even experience some satisfaction, but the activity itself brings no visible joy, just total concentration. It's easy for adults to overlook the exertion that goes into young children's play because we sharply distinguish between work—which we think of as carrying out an obligatory chore—and play, which is purely for fun. And most of us don't think of play as educational because it usually bears little resemblance to what's taught in school.

Yet it's important for parents to understand and appreciate the value of play. Through these often solitary games, small children teach themselves an impressive array of skills—from physical coordination to counting. And by using make-believe to mimic the actions and behavior of grown-ups, boys and girls slowly begin to understand what it means to be a responsible, cooperative member of society.

During a child's first six to twelve months, she will try to get hold of any object within reach, from a wooden spoon to a rattle to a set of keys. She'll turn it over endlessly, chew on it, bang it on the table, and shake it if it makes a noise. These actions are all serious attempts at exploration and experimentation, not like an adult scientist's peering through a microscope to analyze an intriguing new substance.

By the age of one year, children become fascinated with putting small objects into larger containers and then trying to squeeze larger objects into smaller ones. Pushing a wheeled plaything (or just a cardboard carton) around the house is another activity that may captivate a young child for hours. It can take a child at this age months to discover how to avoid obstacles as she steers her toy around and around banging it into walls and tables. It will also take her months to realize that it's easier to pull big objects than to push them. But the patience and determination that children show in applying themselves to such tasks are proof of what a serious matter play is and what a high priority teaching themselves simple manipulative skills has.

Parents and some professionals have trouble understanding why babies take such a long time to learn some play skills while picking up others with surprising speed. For instance, an adventurous one-year-old might teach herself in a single afternoon how to scramble up a flight of stairs on hands and knees—a feat that takes both coordination and courage. Yet the same child may struggle for days to fit a large triangular block into a small circular hole. As Swiss psychologist Jean Piaget showed in his landmark studies on child development, small children will learn these skills in their own way and at their own pace. It's essential for parents to respect nature's mysterious timetable rather than trying to push a child to master skills before she's ready.

Of course, there are ways for mothers and fathers to participate in a child's play without pressuring her to excel. Games of patty-cake or peek-a-boo are likely to send a one-year-old into peals of gleeful giggles, and a two-year-old may enjoy a drawing session with a parent. These joint activities are fine as long as the parent lets the child take the initiative most of the time; in fact, it pleases a young child to find a parent following her lead. But some parents (and I was one of them) can't resist the temptation to lead the play. They see an opportunity to make a game more elaborate and exciting and they take over. I remember years ago watching my young son as he tried to make a toy locomotive go by pushing it across the carpet. "No, no," I said, "We have to put it on the track, like this." Pretty soon he wandered off to find a new game of his own.

Between sixteen months and two years of age, children start to spend more and more time watching their parents and trying to copy their actions. These boys and girls are fascinated by everyday tasks, from sweeping the walk to driving a car. A two-year-old might devote an entire afternoon in the sandbox preparing a make-believe meal using a spoon to stir "eggs" in a bowl, measuring "salt" and "pepper" into the mixture, pouring water on top. These games are usually solitary; a child of this age might enjoy watching other children play and may copy their play actions, but she won't yet join in cooperative play with another youngster.

Why are children under three years content to play alone? Before that age, children don't feel a strong and generous love for each other or a joy in cooperating. A baby's love is directed primarily toward her parents and is based on dependency. She feels love for those on whom she can rely to give her what she needs, whether it is food, security in a strange place, or comfort when she's hurt.

Consequently, it's often a wasted effort—or even counterproductive—to try to get children to share before the age of about three years. At two, a child is extremely possessive. She knows exactly what belongs to her, and she will guard her playthings passionately lest someone try to take anything away. If she sees another child reaching for her doll she'll shriek, "Mine," and grab it back. If a sibling tries to join her in a game of blocks, she may hoard all of the pieces and refuse any assistance. She may however, enjoy "parallel play" in which she watches what another child is doing and copies the action.

When parents force a child of two years to share her toys with a playmate, the child feels betrayed. Not only does she feel that the other child is trying to steal her things, but her own parents are in on the scheme! As a result, the child may become even more possessive and wary of sharing. But if parents wait patiently until the child shows an interest in playing cooperatively, than it's fine to encourage sharing. The best way to accomplish this is to offer suggestions that make sharing fun. "You pull Charlie in your wagon, and then he'll pull you," a parent might say to her child. Or, "You be the bus driver, and Charlie gets on the bus. Then Charlie is the driver, and you get to go for a ride." If the child rejects the suggestion, then it's best to wait a month longer before broaching the subject of sharing again.

At three and four years old, children may still spend plenty of time playing happily on their own, but they also begin to take pleasure in playing cooperatively with their peers especially if they have had previous opportunities. At the same age, children identify strongly with their parents; they copy their parents' actions, talk like them, and walk like them. The most popular game among children of this age is "house." The boy says to the girl, "I'll be the father and you be the mother and this doll is our baby." Then each child plays his or her part, often for hours. The boy will pretend to go to the office, shop for groceries, or care for the children if his father does; the girl will act out in great detail what her mother does at home or in an outside job, mimicking her words and tone of voice.

In a game of house, a child pretending to be the father may need to soothe a crying baby or help two bickering siblings resolve a conflict; he'll also need to find a way to divvy up the household duties with the mother. And a child playing nursery school teacher might praise her younger sibling for solving a puzzle, or scold him for misbehaving. In these ways, children begin to understand what it means to be a man or a woman, a worker, and a parent. They learn how to be responsible, fair, considerate, and loving, and they develop basic ideals and attitudes that will stick with them throughout their lives.

Unfortunately, in our society—where schooling plays such a prominent role children's upbringing—many parents ignore the great value of play and become concerned with how soon their three- or four-year-old child can learn to read and write and do arithmetic.

Their assumption is that an early academic start will put their child ahead of his peers throughout school and in life. In fact, studies show that while a preschooler who is pushed early may learn fast in the short run, his gains level out only a few years later. Meanwhile the child may fall behind his peers in his social and emotional development.

All too often, when adults see children at a day-care center or nursery school "just playing house" or "just playing store" or "just playing bus," they worry that precious time is being wasted that could more wisely be spent mastering the 3 Rs. But that's putting the cart before the horse. Three- and four-year-olds are naturally drawn to play-acting so that they can understand how to become responsible adults. Children shouldn't interrupt these valuable activities with formal schooling until they're at least in kindergarten—and even then they should be given ample time during the day for make-believe and other games.

There's no harm in responding to a curious four-year-old's questions about what a numeral or letter is called, for instance. What I'm arguing against is pressuring teachers to set up organized programs for teaching the academic subjects to preschoolers.

Through early childhood games, children practice some of the most important skills anyone can ever learn; cooperation, sharing, getting along with and caring for others, learning how to grow into mature men and women, fathers and mothers. These qualities are essential for making the world go around and for helping people become productive and happy in their adult lives. We should be thankful that nature has ordained a time for small children to learn so many valuable skills with such intensity and enthusiasm.

Sibling Rivalry

There are a number of different elements in sibling rivalry. In the first place, we humans belong to one of the "pecking order" species. We naturally and easily watch each other suspiciously not only as children but as adults too, to see whether someone else is getting more than we are, getting more than his share—of attention, of prestige, of pay, of love, of clothes.

You can be sure that if a parent obviously favors one child over another, the less favored one will be aware of this in every cell of his body, in every moment of the day. But I don't mean by this that every parent should love each child in exactly the same way; that's impossible because every child is different and parents appreciate different qualities in different children in different ways. You love a gentle child for his or her gentleness. You love a boy you call "Butch" or a girl you call a "tomboy" for their casualness and imperturbability. One child may obviously irritate you more than another. But that doesn't mean less love; in fact you may say, "She's just like me; we understand each other; that's our reason we rub each other the wrong way."

I've noticed that the first child is likely to be more rivalrous with the second than the second is with the third, although this is not an invariable happening. One factor here is that the first has had the parents all to himself for several years, so he is not used to sharing their attention; whereas the second and third have had to share the parents from the start. And the first overcomes some of the bitterness of his rivalry by assuming that he is one of the grown-ups in the family. He takes a condescending attitude toward the baby: "Look, Mom, what a mess he makes with his cereal!"

The first child is apt to be sensitive in human relations, to hang back when playing with other children, to get his feelings easily hurt when they are thoughtless or mean. By contrast the second child is apt to greet a strange child with immediate pleasure which tends to bring out the friendliness of the stranger. Another aspect of this increased sensitivity among some first children is a lowered self-esteem which may be a problem throughout life.

Where loving parents see the social sensitivity of their first child they are apt to assume that it is all a disadvantage. But it isn't. Because of his sensitivity, he is more likely to identify with the problems of others and to make a career in one of the so-called helping professions: teaching, social work, nursing, psychology, or medicine. And because of his seriousness, he is more apt to make a success of it. First children tend to get high grades in school and they are more serious minded. A majority of parents appreciate these qualities.

Quite aside from the special problems and advantages of the heightened jealousy of the first child are the problems connected with sibling rivalry in general, whether it's the first or the fifth child.

From the perspective of parents, I think that this kind of quarreling does as much as anything to spoil the pleasure of parenthood. In some otherwise healthy families, it is continuous and loud enough to be audible everywhere in the house—and sometimes it carries over to the neighbor's house!

The first time I realized how much the parents' attitude could contribute to rivalry, I was amazed. A couple, who had three young boys in a constant uproar of complaining, shouting, and snatching, were offered a two-week winter vacation by the grandparents. The boys were not included in the invitation. The devoted mother, who telephoned home every night of her absence expecting to hear the sitter's complaints about constant fights and her threats to quit the job, heard only perfect reports. When the parents did return, they saw for themselves how the boys curled up on the sofa to be read to and how quietly they played. Yet the sitter, who was middle-aged, was not at all intimidating or even strict. She was agreeable in manner with the boys.

The mother was devoted to her children, but she was often irritable and had a defeated attitude in dealing with the boys. She complained to them and scolded them a lot, but you could see that she didn't expect at all to change them. I felt that the messages they got from her were to deal with each other with irritation and accusations, to hope to get their mother to side with whomever was the loudest complainer in each quarrel, but not to expect it. The mother and her three sons were defeated before they started each fight. Nobody was in control.

The sitter and the boys created a different situation.

The boys knew that the sitter was in charge and steered things in the way she wanted them to go. But she didn't have to get irritable or angry; she could stay calm and affectionate because she had confidence in her self and her child care skills. She was probably brought up by a calm, self-assured, affectionate mother.

I don't mean to say that everyone follows the pattern of their managerial parent to the letter. Various factors play a part. One child is like his parent in one respect, another may succeed in turning out the exact opposite at least in that respect. But every father and mother is influenced in one way or another by the way he or she was raised by his or her own parents.

How do you help your children to avoid or minimize the pain of excessive rivalry, help yourself to avoid the constant irritation, help your grandchildren to avoid making each other miserable, and when they are grown, from being jealous spouses, jealous fellow workers?

To keep a first child from believing he's the only pebble on the beach, I'd take him, as soon as he can walk, to play where there are other children his age, whether it's in a playground, a neighbor's backyard, or a preschool. He won't learn "cooperative play" as yet; that comes at about three years of age. But he'll get experience with what's called "parallel play" and realize how many other children there are in the world and that they grab and pull his playthings without ceremony and want to take them home. At the same time, parallel play gives a child the experience of playing near other children, to observe the responses of others.

I think it's wise not to interfere right away when your one- or two-year-old gets into a tussle as long as he is not being beaten up by an older or more aggressive child. If you do have to interfere, do it in a matter-of-fact spirit as if that is life; just break it up. In other words, do not act as if the persecutor is a fiend from whom you must rescue your helpless child. Let him learn gradually to fight his own battles as long as they are not too one-sided. If your child gets bullied regularly in one location, see if you can find another place where there are no bullies.

In handling the quarrels between two of your own children, I think it's wiser not to search for who started it. Children never admit they started it. Each one digs up an episode that he thinks justified his own retaliation. What this really means is that each one in his quarrels hopes to win the parent's approval of his behavior and the parent's condemnation of his opponent. My mother always expected that her children would have table manners, as did her mother. I can remember clearly how I would watch my siblings at the table, and when the opportunity came, I would say to our mother, "Betty is chewing with her mouth open." My mother would say, "Betty, chew with your mouth closed," and I would rack up a point for myself, feeling quite righteous. What a snob and fuddy-duddy!

I used to assume that the quarrels of sibling rivalry were inevitable, and advised parents to put up with them as one of the prices of parenthood. I definitely disagree with that attitude now. There is too much hatred and violence in our country and around the world and it's getting worse. We will destroy ourselves if we don't get the violence under control and substitute consideration, kindness, and affection. I believe that we can start at home in our relationships with our children and others.

Children pattern themselves after their parents and other adults. Parents must remember that their children are watching them as many hours as they are together. They should strive to set a good example of respect for each other and respect for their children. Not more punishment, but more respect.

When one of their children begins to quarrel or be mean, I now believe that parents should stop what they are doing, move in close to the child, look him squarely in the eye and say quietly and in a kindly spirit, "When you do something like that to your sister, it makes her unhappy and it makes me unhappy. I would like you to think of that the next time." This is much more effective in the long run than shouting at the child or slapping him, both of which send the wrong message.

How to Help a Child Who Isn't Popular

I'll start with the basic question of how to avoid raising children who are less sociable than average.

We should recognize first that children are born with quite different personalities. One is distinctly outgoing, energetic, relatively insensitive to hurts of the physical or social kind, likely to make a go of any situation. At the opposite extreme is the cautious, quiet, sensitive individual whose feelings are easily hurt and who then pulls back into a shell. As a parent you can modify these types somewhat, but you can't turn one into the other.

Many first children are less sociable than average, though they may make compensations as they grow older. (As you may suspect from my sympathy with them, I was the oldest.) They are apt to assume from infancy that they are small adults. They model themselves exclusively on their parents because there are no older children to copy. So they tend to be more serious minded, more mature, more striving, more self-conscious than second and third children. They may be less carefree and playful, so sociability does not come as easily.

When a first child, let's say it's a girl, begins to be around other children, beginning at two years and extending to six years of age, she is not prepared for their noisiness, their roughness in play, their tendency to grab. They scare her, make her shrink back. She's used to the polite and considerate nature of her parents and their friends who compliment her, make up to her, and make no demands on her. She may feel at least a little suspicious and resentful of other children. This will show in her face and manner and put the other children off. So it's a slightly vicious circle.

Before we go on to the ways to help children who lack popularity we should ask how valuable it is anyway. I have the impression that a majority of us Americans put a higher value on sociability than the people of other countries I've visited. We are inclined to think that everyone should make a great effort to be likable. We look askance at loners and eccentrics, whereas in England and France, for instance, they are apt to get full respect, and the child or adult who is withdrawn or pompous may be appreciated.

Some of the world's greatest writers, artists, composers, and scientists have been shy, relatively unsociable people. It seems that their social isolation, their inability to throw themselves into the rough-and-tumble of childhood funneled a lot of their energy and creativity into some special interest or hobby in childhood, and into their chosen field later. They can be loving, responsive people with their intimate relatives and friends, as adults. But this doesn't mean that parents have to choose between popularity and achievement for their children—they can aim for a reasonable balance.

I think of two ways to keep the first child from getting off on the wrong foot. The first is for the parents to try to avoid putting her in the center of the stage from the start. This is hard to do, for it's natural for parents to be exceedingly wrapped up in their first, to be tremendously proud of her smallest accomplishments, to make up games to play with her all day, to greet her enthusiastically each time she creeps or toddles into view, to hang over her protectively whenever she climbs. It's normal and helpful and important for parents to do all these things in moderation. But the first child often gets five times as much attention as the second child, five times as much as is necessary. So she may grow up expecting a great deal of attention and admiration, feeling resentful if it's not forthcoming, disliking other children when they don't give it. She is apt to feel quite hurt by the arrival of a baby brother or sister. The second or third child is more apt to be left to his own devices a greater part of the time. But when he's sociable, he takes the initiative to approach a parent or child, and lays on the charm. He learns ways to be sociable by working at them actively and getting the rewards. However, I don't want you to get the idea you should try to ignore your first. It's a matter of allowing him to take the initiative half the time.

Another, highly important, way to promote sociability is to take children to where other young children play—playgrounds, parks, backyards—from the time they can walk, and perhaps attend a nursery school or day-care center by the age of three years. (I don't mean that all children should attend nursery school, only that it is a good way to learn sociability.) In such groups children get used to rough-and-tumble play, learn to enjoy it, before they are old enough to become self-conscious, or get hurt feelings. When I've suggested that parents search for a place where young children and mothers congregate, they sometimes say, "There are no small children in our neighborhood." That's too bad, but it's not a sufficient excuse. You just have to search farther.

Once again, I want to make the point that there's not much cooperative play or generosity with toys before three years. So parents shouldn't try to force it;

that only makes a two-year-old more possessive of his things. He feels that everybody, including his parent, is trying to rob him of what's his.

In a good nursery school or day-care center with trained teachers (not more than five children per adult) who are concerned primarily with helping individual children meet small crises rather than just keeping order, the children are constantly learning how to get along with each other. This is because each child is regularly surrounded by others, fascinating cooperative play is always going on, and children of this age become fond of each other and so want to get into friendly play. One of the teacher's main jobs is to distract children from quarrels, help them to appreciate each other, share playthings while playing together. Parents, just as well as nursery school teachers, can say, "First you pull Charlotte in the wagon, then Charlotte can pull you. That's fun."—an exciting discovery at three years old.

When children get to elementary school age, they become more sensitive to criticism from other children, more unhappy about not being popular. Parents have real opportunities to foster popularity at this age period. They can invite other children, one at a time (two is company, three's a crowd that tends to split into two and one), for treats such as picnics, trips to the museum, zoo and the beach, attendance at movies, plays, the circus, sports events, a fishing or camping trip, even an overnight trip to another city. Children like to be invited to family meals at a restaurant or at the home of a friend.

In offering experiences like these you are in a sense buying popularity for your child, and bought popularity doesn't last long. However, you are operating on the assumption that your child has appealing qualities to offer but hasn't had a chance to show them because he or she is shy and on the defensive, or because the cliquish nature of the gang hasn't given your child a chance. The period from about eight to thirteen years old is noted for its cliques and its discrimination against newcomers and other outsiders.

Parents can also gently, sympathetically, point out to the selfish child that other children will enjoy playing with him more if he is generous—and that he will feel good too. This works better than scolding. Parents can encourage a timid child to ask in a friendly way for what he wants.

Adolescents are more complicated. They are apt to be so self-conscious, so afraid of criticism from the group that they don't want their parents to interfere in any way in their social life. On the other hand, most of them are so ready and eager for intense relationships, first with those of their own sex, that they manage to find one or two kindred souls with whom they share some special interest, and are thus able to overlook their lack of popularity with the larger group.

Some children experience an unusually high degree of unpopularity. These may be a distinctly aggressive child, the withdrawn child who has no friends at all, the boy who shuns other boys and wants to play only with girls, the child who always seems to get persecuted, and the child who is miserably unhappy about his unpopularity. These children should benefit from counseling. Beginning with your child's pediatrician, family physician, or nurse practitioner is a good way to start the assessment.

As parents, most of us would probably like to have children who are well liked by many, who have half a dozen really close friends, and who also have solid qualities of character. But we can't have everything in each child. For the long pull, I would give the highest priority to solid qualities and absorbing interests, combined with the desire and ability to find at least one satisfying friendship. Having lots of friends and being unusually popular would be a nice extra if a child or adolescent happened to be able to achieve that, but it is certainly not essential for a good life. In fact, some of the teenagers who are unusually popular because they are good-looking, self-assured and affable, poop out later because they don't have qualities that give long-term meaning to life.

And a majority of the individuals who are shy in childhood outgrow this later and become satisfyingly sociable.

Peer Pressure in Adolescence

Peer pressure in adolescence is a frightening thing for parents—as well as for the children—at this period in history when the young are challenging so many basic values: demanding the right to sexual freedom at younger and younger age periods and becoming involved increasingly in pregnancies, experimenting with drugs and alcohol even when very young.

Peer pressure can be amazingly powerful. It can get girls, who love and crave their sleep, out of bed at 5:30 on dark winter mornings in order to wash, dry, and set their hair. It can make natural students ashamed of the good grades they are getting. It can persuade boys and girls who are basically law-abiding and parent-respecting to use alcohol and pot, at least experimentally.

There are really two aspects to peer pressure. One, which you might call active—when another child applies pressure to your child, with promises of pleasure or with taunts about your child being a scaredy cat. Kids do this to other kids because they will feel more justified in their own behavior if they can get other kids, especially strictly brought-up ones, to join in doing the forbidden act.

The passive side of peer pressure—and it's the more powerful—is your child's need to conform to what the others are doing.

Before we assume that peer pressure is always the enemy of parents and the enemy of civilization, we ought to try to look at it objectively. It is so strong and universal that it must have a serious purpose. I believe it's related to rebelliousness against parents, which is designed to make you want to leave your home eventually, get a job, get married, and start a family of your own; otherwise it would be more practical to remain in childlike dependence on parents for life. But we human beings are belongers. We can't give up one form of dependence, in a stage of transition like adolescence, without grasping for another.

You can see this in a humorous way when Americans traveling in foreign lands in the summer and feeling homesick for their own kinds of food, customs, and language, are overjoyed when they find other Americans though they may have nothing else in common. You can see it in a most serious form in the occurrence of suicide in adolescence among those who haven't found a group to belong to or beliefs to sustain them. Many adolescents join a church, a few become fanatics. So clinging to your peers is not the invention of the devil. It's a sort of mental-health measure to keep you from feeling lost. Later, after you settle down into a job and start a family of your own, you'll be able to relax this slavish dependence on acceptance by your peers because you'll feel like a full-fledged member of the whole community or society.

We can get a perspective by realizing that some of the past teenage customs supported by peer pressure that raised parental alarm in earlier decades didn't wreck the society or ruin all the young. In fact they seem pretty tame now—the hippie mode of dressing that revolutionized personal appearances in the 1960s, the miniskirts of the 1970s, and the rebellion of the flappers against corsets and formal manners at dances in the 1920s; even smoking by women was considered shocking then.

Every historical period of relaxed standards is followed sooner or later by a period of formality and tightening of discipline, in which adolescent peer pressure plays a part, too.

Today in many parts of the country there is a swing back to clothes that are attractive and more formal. Eventually it will affect all teens. Hollywood moviemakers report that adolescents are turning away from films showing the explicit details of sexual intimacy and prefer, as they sit with their dates and among their peers, a more sentimental and veiled view of love. I'd say that, having won their right to see everything, they show they have taste and tender feelings underneath, like people in other age groups. And it is reported that the use of pot by the young is declining.

How can parents maintain their maximum influence on their children during their rebellious years, so that the children are least likely to be thrown off course by peer pressures that are harmful?

The first thing they should realize is that their adolescent children's main stabilizer is not the parents' vigilance or rules or warnings or threats. It's the children's admiration for their parents, their desire to grow up to be like their parents which set their course way back in earlier childhood, particularly in the three to six year period. From six or seven years onward, children don't think of those ideals as coming from their parents; they think of them as their own.

The most effective method of reaching teenagers is

through parental attitudes and manner of talking. But this is not easy. The easy thing for parents is to get bristly and antagonistic, or to speak of their age and experience, or to interrupt impatiently and speak con- descendingly. Young people want most of all to be treat- ed like adults; and while that's not always possible, since they don't have the experience and parents have the responsibility, it's worth trying to keep to the adult-to- adult level as much as possible. This means making yourself available when they want to talk, drawing them out rather than interrupting, listening thoughtfully and understandingly ("I see what you mean," or "I often had that feeling"), being honest, showing a sense of humor, trying to be relaxed.

Adolescents are trying to find out all they can about life and they are interested in hearing adults as well as their peers. Underneath they really want to know, and deserve to know, what their parents think about dating, falling in love, sex, marriage, drugs, alcohol, tobacco, education, various occupations, world events, politics, etc. But they are wary about asking their parents' opin- ions for fear the parents will come out with arbitrary and moralistic rules. They don't want their parents to preach at them or act as if the parents know they are right just because they are older. It's all right for parents to express their opinions vigorously, colorfully, as long as they don't claim superior judgment because they are parents. No pomposity. Just because teenagers continue to argue their own opinions against their parents' doesn't mean that they haven't been impressed or even won over by their parents' views. Having been at the disadvantage of being younger all these years, they hate to admit that they may be mistaken.

No matter how opposed you may be to some specific request, it's important to show a general attitude of confidence in the good intentions and good sense of your children. For if they feel that you have no trust in them, then they say, "What's the use of trying to do right by them, when they don't believe you?"

Can't parents ever put their foot down and make a ruling on some request? Of course they have to, from time to time, especially if they have a teenager who is always testing the limits, always thinking up rash things to propose. Then the parent can say, in the end, something like, "I hate to be a killjoy or responsible for your safety and good reputation. If you should get into trouble because I've let you do something that I think is dangerous, I'll blame myself as a parent, and the parents of all your friends will blame me too."

But if you have generally been a responsible parent who respects your kids' judgment, you can count on them to be persuaded by your sensible opinions most of the time. Try to keep your arbitrary decisions down to a minimum.

Sometimes teenagers will cook up a wild plan such as fifteen-year-olds gathering Saturday night at a notorious roadhouse that has had violence at times. They may not be really sure that they want to do it, but they like to think that they have the courage. When a parent, after hearing them out, says, "Sorry, that's out," they may be relieved to have the decision taken out of their hands.

Certainly it's the parents' right and obligation to draw up some rules of behavior ahead of time, preferably in the early teens when children are still used to controls. I would list: no driving in a car with a driver who has been drinking at all. Teenagers should tell parents before going out whom they are going with, where they expect to be, when they expect to get home; and then if delayed they should telephone. Parents can make such rules seem reasonable and fair by following them when they go for an adult evening out. No parties in the homes where there are no adults in charge to take responsibility. No staying in motels or hotels.

If your adolescents strongly object to some rule, you can show your desire to be reasonable by saying you'll think it over and perhaps discuss it with the parents of some of their friends. You don't have to believe their statements that "Everybody I know is allowed to do that." They don't mean to lie, but they have to exaggerate in arguing their positions.

A small item: don't try to use teenage slang, teenage expressions, to show that you are companionable. You may not use them correctly; and this effort to be young is usually embarrassing to the young, especially in the presence of their friends.

It may be helpful, though, to talk a little, with humor, about your own youth occasionally—things that embarrassed you about your parents, adventures that scared you, unrealistic demands that you presented to your parents, or peer pressures that you did or didn't yield to. Such confessions show that you were human once and haven't forgotten it. But don't use these recollections to prove that you are always right now—that would block the sense of mutual understanding that you are trying to establish.

Remember that teenagers are always being pulled in two opposite directions: They yearn to be more independent, but underneath they are at least a little scared of succeeding in cutting loose and then having no one to take care of them. A fifteen-year-old girl once came to my office to complain bitterly and lengthily that her parents were keeping her tightly tied to their apron strings. But after a few appointments, she was complaining more about how her mother was neglecting her—for instance, in not making her sandwich and pouring her glass of milk before going out to work, so the girl had to prepare her own lunch on coming home from school. You'll notice that in both complaints it's the parents who are held at fault.

About drugs, alcohol, and tobacco, my own inclination would be not to try to extract promises or lay down rules, because I would be pretty sure they would be broken. Almost all adolescents crave to try these supposed delights at least a few times, as we remember from our own childhood. When the subject comes up sometime in the early teens or even before, because of questions or gossip, I'd talk along the following lines: "All teenagers want to try these at least a few times. I did myself. But tobacco kills many people with lung cancer or heart disease. Alcoholism kills people through liver disease and wrecks families through loss of jobs, brutality, and shame. Most drugs are physically or psychologically addictive. They distract you from studies and other activities at a difficult time in life when you are going through deep changes and having to prepare for college and your life's work. I'd advise you to postpone all of them until you are at a more settled down period, at least eighteen, and know more exactly what you want out of life." I wouldn't say anything that is not scientifically known because teenagers know a lot and lose faith in people who are alarmist or careless with the truth. I'd keep in mind that my advice is much more likely to be adopted if, as a parent talking to my son or daughter, I don't smoke or drink or take any drugs regularly including tranquilizers, sedatives, and stimulants.

I would take comfort from the realization that the children who get into serious trouble with alcohol or drugs are not the sensible children of stable families but the ones who have been visibly troubled for a long time.

Peer pressure to be sexually bold comes to adolescents from those of their own sex who want to relieve their own guilt by persuading all others to do the same things. At other times, peer pressure comes from the opposite sex, especially boys. But both boys and girls may have a particularly strong drive to experiment with seductiveness in the early stages of adolescence before they've gained any confidence in their ability to attract or to perform. At this stage, there may be little or no tenderness, generosity, compatibility or love in these usually brief attractions.

How parents want to guide their children's early approach to sex, love, and future marriage will depend greatly on the parents' own ideas and ideals. Some will encourage early dating, with coaching, teasing, giving parties that include kissing games.

At the opposite extreme are parents who want their children to move slowly and retain some of their inhibitions until they know themselves and have learned from social experiences the characteristics they desire in a person of the opposite sex. They want their children to develop and retain an idealistic, spiritual view of marriage, and to keep sex subordinated to that ideal. They'll encourage their young teenagers to stay in groups when they go to movies, concerts, suppers, dances, excursions, camping trips under supervision in preference to pairing off. They'll realize that their own respect and love for each other will be the strongest influence of all in setting their children's ideals. When conversation in the family turns to sex and marriage, they'll avoid cheap jokes. They'll remind their children—without being stuffy about it—that infatuation is exciting but usually not lasting, that the right marriage can be endlessly satisfying and inspiring; but it takes a long time to be sure of the right person, and marriage requires continual cultivation, devotion, thoughtfulness, like a garden or a highly creative career.

Compare and Despair

Some children are unhappy because they think they are not as popular or as successful or as good-looking or as skilled as their friends or their brothers and sisters.

Until I worked as a counselor at a home for handicapped children during my summer vacation from college in the 1920s, I'd always assumed, in my youthful innocence, that adults and children would be realistic about their strong points and their handicaps. I'd assumed that they would be a little sad if they had a small handicap, very sad if they had a serious one, and exceptionally happy if they were extraordinarily beautiful or popular or athletic.

You can imagine my surprise when I found that though all children at the home had a serious physical disability, some of them were on the morose side, some were average in mood, and others were as cheerful and optimistic about life as if they had been perfect specimens.

After this truth had sunk in I realized that, among people who have no noticeable physical defect, there is a similar variation in mood, from glum to enthusiastic.

By the time I was a practicing pediatrician, I got additional slants. I recall being consulted about an attractive teenage girl who was sure that her looks were ruined and that she was doomed to be shunned by girls and boys because she had freckles on her nose, which she would gaze at sadly every time she got near a mirror.

I also came to realize that an important factor—perhaps the most important—in how a child feels about a handicap, great or small, is how the parents feel about it. I remember a mother who, when she found that her daughter had been born with an almost total impairment of hearing (which meant that even with the best of special training and schooling she would also have a noticeable speech defect) went into a depression and largely rejected the child from that time onward, with serious emotional consequences for the child, too. The parents, because of their feelings of hopelessness, neglected the opportunities for technical aids, special training, and special schooling.

I saw a contrasting situation with another girl, also born with almost complete hearing loss, who was sixteen years old when I first knew her. Though her speech was hard to understand until you became accustomed to it, she was happy, she was high spirited, she was attractive and she was really popular. Her parents had been able, with the help of good counselors, to outgrow their initial shock and dismay, to overcome the guilt that is common in such situations, and to accept and love the child as she was. They had followed professional advice and seen to it that she had all the advantages of technical aids, special training, and special schooling to enable her to make the most of her education.

Children in their earliest, most formative years develop their evaluation of themselves not by comparing themselves with others, as they will do later, but by sensing what their parents feel about them. Children whose parents consider them basically bad or basically good, dull or bright, homely or beautiful, uninspired or talented, tend to accept these judgments, whether they are expressed openly or harbored secretly.

A potent way in which children's self-assurance is undermined is when parents scold frequently, let their anger show freely, or merely look disapproving a lot of the time. The effect on children, especially when they are young, is a chronic subconscious or conscious fear that the parent will stop loving them. People of all ages need and yearn to be loved. But children, realizing that they are utterly dependent on their parents for every kind of care, dread the possible end of loving much more than adults do. Yet the implied withdrawal of love, when disapproval is steady or frequent, is probably the most common means that parents use to pressure their children to conform, and it always undermines self-confidence to a degree.

A similar but less frequent way in which parents may make their children sensitive and insecure about themselves is by telling them that other people won't like them if they misbehave or show certain traits. My mother used this leverage on her six children and it certainly made us painfully self-conscious about the impression we made on others.

Another factor that makes for self-consciousness and self-doubt is the comparison of one child with another that most parents find themselves doing, even parents who disbelieve in comparisons and competition. For most parents themselves were compared in childhood and it's hard to break a pattern that you were brought up in. "Why don't you practice piano conscientiously, like your sister does?" or "Harry Jenkins' mother tells me the reason he earns such good grades is because he does two hours of homework every night" or "Rose Gibbons is a beautiful child; she'll never have to worry about getting a good job or a good husband." Each little comparison may seem unimportant by itself but the accumulation of them throughout childhood is apt to give a child a conviction that she will be constantly compared throughout life, in our highly competitive society.

Another factor I'd like to mention is inborn temperament. Studies have shown that babies are born with quite different temperaments and that these tend to persist, to one degree or another, depending on life's experiences. The child who is born active, extroverted, physically fearless, is much less likely to worry about any inadequacies, real or imagined, than the child born sensitive and cautious.

Sometimes when a child keeps complaining to her parent that she is less attractive or less successful she is asking, without being conscious of it, for reassurance, not just that her qualities are good but that she is loved for herself.

What can you do for the self-doubting child? I feel that prevention is even more important than the cure.

The first step would be to try to treat your first child in the less preoccupied, less interfering, less worried manner as you will probably treat your second. Let her amuse herself for part of her wakeful periods. Let her develop her own caution—about climbing on the sofa and other physical challenges where a fall would not be dangerous. Take her, as soon as she can walk, to a playground or other neighborhood gathering place where there are other children of her age and abilities, and let her learn to fight some of her own battles, as long as she's not being badly or chronically outfought.

The fewer children there are in your own neighborhood, the more value there will be in her learning sociability in a good nursery school or day-care center, from the age of three years.

In managing and controlling a child at home, try hard to deal in cheerful positives rather than prohibitions, scolding, and shaming: "We hold hands when we cross the street." "Charlie wants to use your tricycle for a few minutes, then you can use it again." "If you don't like a food, you don't have to eat it. Just leave it on your plate." "The baby loves you. Pat him gently."

If your child is already comparing herself unfavorably with others, try to avoid an argumentative tone. Let yourself go with warm and friendly compliments—about the specific areas in which she says she is lacking, as long as the compliments are not grossly untrue. Then go on to compliment her for other good qualities, too. End up with a beaming, sparkly-eyed declaration of your love for her as a person.

If she wants to go back to complaining or belittling herself, be patient, hear her out, express your sympathy with her unhappiness ("I can see how upsetting it would be for you to think you are not beautiful") without admitting that you share her judgment. Avoid impatience and a strained tone which, in her unhappy mood, she will interpret as a lack of sympathy, a lack of love. Try to act relaxed, confident of your parenting, and affectionate. Repeat again how much you love her.

If she persists in self-belittling, after you have run out of positive things to say, you can try to break her pessimistic spell by changing the subject altogether and suggesting a treat—a meal at a restaurant or a trip to the ice cream store.

If your child has usually been as cheerful as the average child and then slips into a persistent mood that is distinctly self-critical and sad, she may be developing a real depression, with at least a slight risk of suicide. In this situation, your child needs to be under the care of a mental-health professional.

The Neighbors' Kids

There were problems with the neighbors' children in most of the places in which we lived when we were raising two sons. And when I was in pediatric practice, parents often came with similar problems.

Most difficult to deal with is the neighborhood meanie who bullies younger children. Bullies rarely take on children their own size. He may physically hurt his victims—who tend to be the gentler, more sensitive kinds—but more often he just threatens and teases. He is usually a genius in detecting children who are teasable or easily frightened and will keep after them until they run home in tears. It makes me angry just to think of them, since I was sometimes a victim, too, in my childhood.

What's a good parent to do? Least likely to work, in my experience, is to complain to the bully's parents. They are often rather belligerent people—that's how they made their son into a meanie—and they may turn on you harshly, defend their son, and tell you to mind your own business. Go out and scold the boy, yourself? It may work. But its weakness is that it teaches your child that he can't take care of himself, that he needs your protection. Most constructive, if it will work, is to tell your child that the bully only likes to tease if he can get the other child upset, so it's smart to try to pay no attention, just go on playing. That's true enough in theory but it's hard for a smaller, more timid child to carry out.

The safest first step, as a parent, is to approach the bully in a friendly way. If you can give him the benefit of the doubt by assuming that he wouldn't really hurt anyone, explain to him that, when he teases or pretends that he is going to do something mean, it scares a small child who doesn't realize that it's only teasing. So you are asking him, one older person to another, for his understanding and cooperation. It's not a bad idea for the parent to stick around for a while after a talk with the bully—not in a suspicious but in a very friendly spirit—perhaps getting into a game they are playing, to show that the parent is a nice person but is also closely in touch with the situation, not far away.

A further approach, that may sound strange to you, is for you to try to make closer friends with the bully—invite him over, give him snacks, ask him to meals, or on excursions. Make conversation and draw him out. You may be able, with your kindness, to evoke the kind side of his personality—if he has any. Of course you can't do this effectively if you consider him repulsive. But remember that he must be the victim of some kind of open or subtle bullying at home, so that you can feel sympathetic, as a pediatrician or child psychiatrist would. Even if you don't draw out his better nature, he may not feel as free as before to persecute your child.

But can you do anything from the beginning to help prevent your child from becoming the overly sensitive, easily victimized one? I think so. The sensitive child may have been born with a sensitive temperament from the beginning. Or he may have grown up at the center of the family stage with two kind parents who've had a spotlight on him, beamed on him, given him anything reasonable that he wants, and generally been cordial and polite to him. If he has had little contact with other children until he's four or five or six years old, he'll find them rough, grabby, noisy, and inconsiderate by comparison, really quite intimidating. By contrast, other children are thicker-skinned, tougher by a natural process, much less likely to be socially self-conscious or to get hurt feelings when not in center stage. When challenged or attacked by another child, even one considerably larger, these children are apt to stand their ground or fight back without any thought for the consequences.

So my idea is to get every child used to the rough-and-tumble, the give-and-take of play with other children, beginning as soon as he can walk.

Now suppose the shoe is on the other foot and a neighboring parent complains to you that your child is making her child miserable. The only course, it seems to me, is to express genuine regret and promise sincerely to take up the matter with your child. If it turns out to be some misunderstanding on the neighbor's part, no harm is done. But if your child directly or indirectly admits bullying, I wouldn't jump on him, but I'd explain how meanness hurts another child's feelings and suggest that he be extra kind to help heal those feelings. If you've suspected for some time that your child has become more aggressive than normal, presumably because he is upset about something, consult the school people and then, if indicated, your child's pediatrician, family physician, or nurse practitioner.

A very different problem, if you are a person who is naturally hospitable and friendly with children, is having your house or apartment full of the neighbors' children, all day and even into the night. You suspect that some of them are not very welcome at home and so they flock to the place of an adult who's warmhearted and friendly.

It's your privilege to entertain as much or as little as you wish. You have to remember that many children, especially the more aggressive ones, are not sensitive to a polite adult's gentle hints, such as "Your parents may be worried," or "It must be your suppertime at home." If they give you a confidently negative answer, you have to say in a friendly but firm tone, "Now, everybody has to go home!" You may need to add, "Don't come in the morning until ten o'clock" or "Don't come back until I invite you." And then, when several eager faces appear at 7:45 A.M., don't be bashful about saying, "No, we aren't ready for visitors yet. Don't come back until ten." An adult might get hurt feelings from such a pronouncement, not children.

You are entitled to have control over your own backyard, too. I think that parents who want to keep track of their young children should be glad that the other children want to play there. That was my possessive mother's idea. She filled the backyard with a sand-box, a three-seated swing, a seesaw, a simple merry-go-round, and a "jouncing board" (a long, wide sturdy board between two supports). She wanted to oversee and control her own children so she made the backyard inviting to the whole neighborhood, and it worked.

If older meanies or destructive or foul-mouthed types arrive in your yard, or if ordinary, careless children trample your flowers and treat the playthings roughly, I'd advise always using first the friendly explanation of why this behavior upsets the smaller or more timid children, or of how hard you've worked on your garden, hoping to enlist the sympathy of the children. Then stay in the yard for a while or even join in the play. This usually is enough to make the bullies and the vandals leave, because there isn't enough left to do that interests them.

I'd avoid getting agitated or angry if you possibly can. Tough kids enjoy stirring up the adults who fly off the handle. And normal children like to gossip about those particular people in the neighborhood who are always so cross and ready to scold that they are considered witches and ogres. In small, hard-to-detect ways, children enjoy making a little trouble for such people and treating their children as natural enemies. If your yard should ever be invaded by a tough, destructive youngster, I think it's better to just call the police than to holler at them in frustration.

What do you do if you get robbed or vandalized and suspect certain teenagers from the neighborhood? If I had pretty good proof, my own preference would be to speak to the parents of the boys and let them handle it from then on, if they accept responsibility. If they deny the evidence or if I have no proof, I'd simply do nothing or notify the police. In many such minor cases the police, if they find evidence, will only lecture boys for their first offense, and this is often enough to scare them out of further experiments with lawlessness.

A really sticky problem with neighboring teenagers is when your daughter decides she must give a party, not for a few friends but for two or three dozen. She says she doesn't want you to be there; it would spoil the party and embarrass her so much that she'd rather not have it. What often happens is that, in addition to the invited guests, there come nearly as many uninvited classmates, and some of them may be drunk, noisy, and with a chip on their shoulders.

My feelings—and I'll be outvoted by all teenagers and many parents—is that parents should be in the house if not on view during parties, up until their children are at least eighteen years old. Then if things begin to get out of hand, the parents are entitled to appear, despite the daughter's or son's disapproval, not to read the riot act but to circulate in a friendly spirit among the guests. This in itself will have a calming, civilizing effect on the party.

Another solution is to urge your teenager to have several separate parties over a period of time with six or eight friends, at home or in a restaurant. These are unlikely to go haywire.

Before ending I want to get back to a general principle of how you make your decisions stick, with preschoolers, elementary schoolers, or teenagers, whether neighborhood children or your own.

The problem gets greater as the children grow older. It's worse than useless to make any threat that you can't or won't carry out. Basically you have to count on what I'd call your moral authority in controlling the neighborhood children, just as you do with your own. You have to have a conviction that you have the right to insist on good behavior. That's what carries your conviction over to the children and convinces them that they should and must go along. This is hard for those parents to believe who were themselves brought up with angry shouts and threats and blows, because their parents had no confidence that there was anything else to count on. But having known dozens of children who were brought up by moral authority alone (with no physical punishment), I can testify that it is more convincing and effective than any threats or spankings.

Your moral authority with the neighborhood children will be reinforced if, after having made a firm request, you stay with them for half an hour to be sure it is carried out. You don't have to be disagreeable. You can be friendly but firm.

6

Education

What Is Education?

Education is not one thing, one process. Memorizing the multiplication tables is basically different from writing interesting compositions, from safe auto driving, from understanding physics, from speaking a foreign language.

To get a sense of learning as a natural process, we can back away for a minute from the many modern technologies that children and youth are expected to study, and see what goes on in nonindustrial societies where the men all have one occupation such as fishing or hunting and the women harvest food, cook, make the clothes, oversee the children.

In infancy, children are driven by instinct to explore and manipulate and test their skills. In their second and third year they are copying parents' activities that are within their understanding and capability—for example, increasingly complex talking, feeding, and brushing teeth.

From three to six years old, they identify intensively with their parents, who love them and whom they adore. They identify predominantly with the parents of the same sex, wanting to be just like her or him, playing at being woman or man, mother or father, practicing their occupations as well as they understand them, their interests and behavior and mannerisms. It's primarily an emotional drive and it's a strong one. The parents set the examples and the children do the work of learning, by patterning themselves after the parents. That's the natural process of education.

Now education is incredibly complex and many sided, but I believe that it will still be most strongly motivated by a warm, mutually respectful relationship between teacher and student, especially in the elementary and high school years. By the time students are in the university most of them are sufficiently self-motivated to be able to apply themselves despite large classes and impersonal instructors.

As civilizations developed and as records and technical information were preserved, the ability to transmit skills and knowledge to their children was not possible for most parents. Schools were set up in which people with special knowledge could teach it to children. Since the subject matter was usually in words and numbers, teaching in past centuries tended to be in the form of the lecture material which children memorized and gave back in recitations. In the Moslem village the pupils, over the years, still memorize the Koran; when that is finally accomplished, they are considered wise men. As knowledge has accumulated over the centuries and millennia, the same pattern has been followed: memorization of lectures or textbooks, recitations, or examinations.

From time to time educational reformers, especially in professional schools such as medical and law, have protested that this approach doesn't necessarily produce knowledge and skills that are usable in real situations. A medical student, for instance, might be able to list the typical symptoms of a disease but not be able to put together the history, the physical examination, and the laboratory test results in such a way as to be able to distinguish a case of one disease from a case of a somewhat similar disease. Or he might have no sense of how to question the patient, how to explain the situation to her, or how to comfort her if the news was bad. The student physician must learn these skills by dealing with live patients under careful supervision.

John Dewey, the philosopher and educator, demonstrated the same principles in elementary and secondary education. Children learn more deeply when they "learn by doing" in a real or simulated life situation. Instead of learning reading in one class period, writing, arithmetic, social studies in other, separate periods, by listening and then reciting, Dewey encouraged participation in a project that is appealing and which links these school subjects. A third grade class may read about Native Americans, write about them, understand what was important to them, and learn how they made their living and migrated before white men came and interrupted their customs. The children may work cooperatively on a model or a mural of a Native American village. A child who is behind in a subject like reading or arithmetic is stimulated to try to catch up by the enthusiasm of the group and of himself for the whole project.

Class work can be "enriched" by extra assignments to challenge the interest and ability of the advanced pupils, provided the class is small (which all classes should be) and the teacher is well trained. If a child is an advanced reader and the class needs to have some library research done, she can be chosen to go to the library—not by the teacher because this may lead to taunts of teacher's pet, but chosen by the whole class as the best person to help them out.

I believe that human relations should be a part of all education. If a quarrel develops between two elementary school students, the teacher shouldn't try to suppress it or ignore it. She can lead a friendly discussion of how it started and developed, how the two individuals felt, how it can be solved, how it could have been avoided.

By junior high, human relations should include sex education in the broadest sense. Sex education should not be limited to the anatomy and physiology of the body, but should include the spiritual aspects of all boy-girl, husband-wife relationships—the idealization of each other which brings out the best in both, the desire to help, to protest and, most of all, to please and keep on pleasing each other, and later the desire to cherish and raise fine children together. Sex education in this broad sense involves all boy-girl, man-woman relation-ships, including dating and curfew times which are of vital concern, particularly in the early teens, cosmetic and clothes styles, and occupations for men and women. Discussion of such topics should be encour-aged in most school classes from biology to literature and history, allowing students to learn these topics at their own level of development and maturation.

Educators keep lapsing back to what I consider mis-taken concepts such as that learning comes in the form of more work in the classroom, that grades and degrees measure knowledge and competence, that the schools' duty is to bring all the students up to the schools' standards or flunk them, that educational reform in America should consist of raising the school's standards and somehow making the students conform by longer hours or more months of schooling or more homework. Studies have shown that none of these raise performance.

The most serious problem in our schools, I believe, is the high dropout rate among students, especially those from deprived backgrounds, in an increasingly technological society. It can only be solved by providing the most inspiring programs and teachers for the pupils with the lowest motivation, recognizing that, at sixteen years of age as at four, the strongest motivations for learning are the child's feeling of being liked and appreciated by the parent or teacher, wanting to grow up to be a somewhat similar person, and a sense of achieving something everyday!

Raising standards and insisting that each student meet them will only increase the dropout rate.

How do parents get the kind of education they desire for their children? By choosing between schools if they have a choice; by attending parent-teacher meetings, speaking up and backing teachers, principals, and school board members in whom they believe; participating in school board elections, not just by voting but by contributing work and money to their approved candidates; speaking up for higher school budgets when they are justified; expressing their preferences for higher teacher salaries (to keep the best teachers teaching) over funds for new athletic equipment, which can often be raised by other means by sports enthusiasts.

How does a parent help her child who seems to have a problem learning in a particular class? Here's one example that might be a guide in other situations as well. If a sensitive child, especially in first or second grade, is overawed or frightened by a stern-appearing teacher, the parents may be able to help by discussing the problem with the teacher or principal, being careful and tactful not to criticize the teacher but to point out the child's oversensitivity. The parents can help the child by listening sympathetically while at the same time pointing out that the teacher has to use whatever methods she feels are right and that the child will have to learn to get along with difficult people all her life.

Incidental Learning

In our technical, industrial society we think of formal schooling—kindergarten, twelve grades, maybe four or more years of college—as the normal learning process.

But there is another kind of learning that is acquired mainly by emotional identification with an admired person, usually older, most often a parent. This is how children learn in societies that have no schools, which is the situation in many parts of the world. Children and youth without much strain or conscious effort, pick up these capabilities and attitudes. You can see this in its simplest form in the way babies of half a year babble as if they think it's talking. Before a year they can learn to play patty-cake after it is demonstrated, and do it with pride and delight. The one-year-old grabs a spoon away from his parent and clumsily feeds himself. He learns a few words, with which he makes do for nearly a year.

I remember a little girl who, at the age of about a year, when she couldn't yet walk alone, responded to the visit of a neighbor by crawling upstairs, getting a garment out of her open bureau drawer, draping it around her neck, and crawling backward down the stairs to model the creation.

Two-year-olds rapidly pick up hundreds and hundreds of new words every week, and the grammatical sense of how to use them, starting with nouns and names of objects and people, moving on to verbs and very brief sentences.

This kind of learning is much more basic and vital

than school learning. It's how animals learn; they not only are without books, they don't even have words. The young watch carefully their parents, with whom they have an intense, dependent relationship.

More than anything else, young children want to grow up to be like their parents. This is how they learn how to get along with people—in marriage, in social life, in their adult jobs. It's not "incidental" learning, it's the most basic, valuable kind of learning that exists. When we try to ignore it, we make all kinds of mistakes, both as parents and as teachers in schools.

Now for some more examples: Boys learn how to be men, how to walk as a man, have the tone of voice of a man, enjoy male friendships, by watching their fathers—and older brother, if any. A good learning relationship depends on a father loving and enjoying his young son; that's how the boy is able to respond by wanting to be like his father. He wouldn't want to be just like a father who didn't show him any affection or didn't even pay much attention to him.

Years ago I watched an example of how a four-year-old girl identifies with her mother. The mother was teaching her four-year-old how to give a bath to a doll, undressing it, bathing it, drying it, diapering it, dressing it, putting it to bed. At every step she repeated the question: "See how I did it, dear? Watch me carefully, dear." Finally she stepped back and passed the job to her daughter's friend, who tried to follow the directions. But the four-year-old soon interrupted, "No, dear, not like that. Now watch me more carefully, dear." Whose overbearing condescending manner is this? Of course, it's the four-year-old's mother's, and the child has learned it exactly by four years of age. You can be quite sure that when she is twenty-four years old and has a child, she will still have the bossy, condescending manner that she had at four. She has already become a mother in her mother's pattern by four years of age.

My mother, who feared almost nobody, had a real horror of drunks. She never talked about it to her children; but I can still remember vividly how her hand tightened on mine, when I was four or five years old and we happened to meet a drunk on the sidewalk downtown. It took me twenty years to outgrow that uneasiness.

Children are most eager to observe people at their occupations and to imagine themselves performing them. Children spend a lot of time "playing house" which really means acting out their parents' roles as they have observed them. The boy pretends to say good-bye to his "wife" in the morning, taking or giving instructions, driving away. If the mother goes out to work, her daughter does likewise, perhaps dropping the children at the day-care center. When both parents participate in child care at home, the children take turns instructing or scolding the doll or younger child they are using in their family play. It is revealing and sometimes embarrassing to parents to observe their children's picture of parental behavior.

Boys and girls watch the activities of men and women doing visible outdoor work (it's more fascinating than "going to the office") such as driving a bus, operating a backhoe, or giving a shot in a physician's office.

The best way to build a desire in young children to go to school later themselves and to be able to read to themselves someday is by reading to them regularly. Parents can begin this process by reading to their children at the earliest possible age—beginning as an infant. Reading books to children teaches the joy and excitement of this shared activity. This is powerful preparation for learning.

As for the harm of pushing formal academic work too early, I'll always remember a movie produced by a psychologist who advocated very early instruction in reading and claimed that he didn't use any pressure. He showed a two-year-old who looked scared as a rabbit that wanted to flee. The boy kept looking around for an escape route but there wasn't any. He mumbled in a timid voice the words that the instructor pointed out. It looked like pressure to me, of a sort that might prejudice him against school learning the rest of his childhood. The scene gave me goose flesh.

It's not just the "good" qualities and attitudes in our parents that we absorb, it's the "bad" ones too. The statistics show clearly that a majority of the men who abuse their wives saw their fathers do the same when they themselves were children. And the parents who abuse their children were abused as children. Even if they consciously disapprove of such behavior, they are apt to slip into it when their patience wears thin.

In closing, I want to discuss the example of how

medical school teaching and residency training in the hospital got tragically off the track in the last part of the nineteenth and the first quarter of the twentieth century. It may seem far away from the question of pre-school learning today, but it is a particularly clear example of the same issue of "incidental" versus school learning in children.

A vital part of medical training is what students and residents pick up, often without realizing it, from faculty members whom they admire and who treat them in a friendly manner. It has been known for centuries that you can't train a medical student by books or lectures alone. In earlier times, when the only science in medicine was anatomy, the student learned that subject by dissecting a cadaver, under supervision. The rest of his teaching consisted of an apprenticeship to a practitioner who took him to see how he practiced medicine, at the bedside, with an attentive, wise manner.

Then in the nineteenth century came the flood of technical sciences that have dominated medical training since then: physiology, biochemistry, microscopic anatomy, pathology (the diagnosis of disease by viewing specimens of blood, urine, feces, spinal fluid, specimens of tissues removed at operations, and by autopsies on the bodies of patients who died). These sciences shifted the diagnosis and treatment of diseases greatly, and also the attitudes of medical teachers. The teachers were scientists now who counted on lectures and the threat of failure at examination time to get the material memorized.

By the end of the nineteenth century, teachers in medical schools were ashamed to make diagnoses such as psychosomatic diseases, when physical symptoms in a patient were often related to stress, anxiety or depression, rather than an infection or some other "medical" cause. All of these conditions, that explain a majority of the causes of visits to the doctor among adult patients then and now, were ignored as imaginary or suspected of being malingering or as self-indulgent "nervousness," not worthy of scientific attention.

When I was in medical school (1925–1929) there was no teaching of the many crucial psychological aspects of medicine, obstetrics, surgery, pediatrics, family relationships or of the doctor-patient relationship. Think of the millions of misdiagnosed, mistreated cases all because the professionals were trying to ignore the so-called incidental learning that occurs naturally when the student gets to know the teacher, feels liked by him or her, and wants to end up with similar attitudes and knowledge. This is in contrast to the student who might identify with some of his teachers, not as warm, compassionate healers, only as impersonal diagnosticians who thought of their patients as "cases."

It has taken half a century to partly eradicate such an attitude.

Competitiveness

Our society is becoming more and more excessively competitive, I feel, from early childhood to the top

executive level of large corporations. Too much competitiveness is contributing to many of our other problems. I don't believe that this has to be. Of course, we
humans belong to one of the pecking order species and
we will always be somewhat rivalrous. You can see it in
the way young children, even in a noncompetitive family, vie for their parents' attention when they are first
learning to swim or in the way they spontaneously start
a running race.

But in a low-competitive society or family the parents
may not comment or even notice such early contests. In
America where competitiveness is valued so highly,
many parents are likely to egg the children on with
shouts and compliments.

I'd say that the rivalry that children feel within themselves, and that is not intended to hurt anyone but is
just for fun, is harmless. It's the rivalry that is stirred up
or spurred on by parents and teachers, or that is meant
to humiliate, that is more likely to distort their sense of
values.

Previously, I gave the example of a psychologist who
claims that he can teach two-year-olds to read and that
he uses no pressure. But a movie of the method shows
him putting considerable pressure on a child who has
the look of a hunted rabbit, darting his eyes to right
and left as if looking for an escape route.

Teachers in day-care centers and nursery schools tell
me that many parents, anxious for their children to
excel, keep asking why their three- and four-year-olds
are not being taught to read and write and learn arith-

metic. The saddest part of this push to make superkids is that no one has proved that very early academic programs produce better readers or more accomplished students later. I suspect that such premature academic work will create in many children tensions and a dislike of all schooling.

At three and four years, children are preparing themselves to be future men, women, fathers, mothers, workers, and cooperative citizens by constantly watching their parents and molding themselves in the parents' image. This is infinitely more important than the 3 R's at this age. In fact, experiments many years ago showed that children learned the 3 R's more quickly and easily with fewer learning problems by beginning at seven years rather than at the traditional six. I see no harm in answering a curious three- or four-year-old's questions about letters or figures. It's parents putting pressure on them that causes tension.

In a majority of our schools and universities, the students gain the impression from their teachers that the goal is not to understand the world and themselves but to get grades and degrees in a competitive system. If the grades are too low, you flunk. If they are unusually high, you will be recognized as superior. Teachers can encourage a better understanding of the community and the larger world through cooperative projects.

Children used to go to summer camp primarily to study nature and to relax in enjoyable activities which they didn't have the facilities or the time for in winter. Now they are more apt to be sent for intensive study of math or computers or to become more "expert" in tennis.

In self-organized, more spontaneous athletics in earlier times, the aim was primarily to have fun and to see how well you could perform. In more recent years the focus, it seems to me, has shifted more and more to winning, with the unspoken assumption that of course you shouldn't expect to have much fun—just gain glory. The coach, who is hired to win, has increasing authority. I know because I participated in eight-oared rowing for three years in college. It was no laughing matter!

Frisbee is my idea of a good game where both sexes can play together and enjoy it. Touch football is another. But you know that if Frisbee or touch football became major sports, coaches would be hired to create winning teams to satisfy the competitive appetites of the alumni.

In towns and small cities, the emotional involvement of most of the male citizens in the success of the high school's football team and in glorifying the outstanding stars is amazing to someone who grew up in a different environment. A majority on the team are levelheaded enough to outgrow the adulation. But I've known individual high school and college stars whose emotional and social growth were stunted at the age level of their athletic triumphs; they never found anything else gratifying enough to challenge them after that. This is exploitation of youth for the competitive excitement of the middle-aged.

The recruiting of high school stars with "athletic scholarships" at colleges, even if they are poor students, seems to me an inducement to cynicism of which we have too much already. I believe that all students who show that they can profit from a university education and who can't afford it should be able to go with expenses paid by government.

I think that organized athletics below the senior high school level is justifiable if the aims are clearly fun and the improvement of skill. But I've heard of games in which parents swarmed out of the grandstand to harass the umpire for a decision they thought unfair. And I've seen a father crash-land on his young son with scorn in the presence of the whole team for a mild blunder, which is humiliating enough to turn a sensitive boy against athletics for life.

Children always feel any kind of stress in their parents, even if they don't always understand it. The excessive competitiveness that many parents transmit to their children is usually not due to the parents consciously trying to stir up ambitiousness to an abnormal degree. It's because the parents themselves are feeling the constant pressure to compete, to get ahead, that so permeates our society that they can't help passing it on. They are usually not even aware that they are under pressure to compete and to make their children compete, because the pressure on them is so persistent that it feels like normal life. It's only when you compare the competitive pressures here with the much lesser tensions in other, simpler societies that you realize how hectically we live.

A father of a teenager who has gotten into trouble

with the law confesses to a counselor that he has been so wrapped up in the corporation he works for, trying so hard to earn an ever higher salary for the supposed benefit of his family and to get to the top for his competitive ego, that he has really lost contact with his children and neglected his wife.

A father says to his son in college, who has become concerned about how government is failing to solve the social and economic problems of the nation, "Don't you worry about politics, son, your job is to get ahead." This advice—to forget politics and the welfare of the nation, and to focus exclusively on "rugged individualism"—is one of the reasons why only half of American adults bother to vote, a poor record for a democracy, and why our government neglects the welfare, the health, and the education of children. Citizens' neglect of politics turns the government over to special interests. This father's advice turns a youth away from the vital democratic action for the common good toward competition for his own advancement.

A majority of men, and now increasing numbers of the women who work, primarily for the satisfactions of a career, assume that their job is the most important aspect of their lives, ahead of family, friendships, and cultural interests such as participation or enjoyment in music, photography, literature, theatricals, games, and nature study.

One way of testing my rash statement is to ask what gets slighted when there isn't enough time for everything? Sick children do have a high priority for professional mothers, but most well children don't have much chance of pulling a professional parent off the job for a treat or to listen to a recital. "Mother (or Daddy) has to work," parents reply. I've listened to children express this dissatisfaction. They complain too about not getting much time in the evenings or on weekends.

Few of the examples I've given of the stirring up of rivalry and competitiveness in childhood and youth by parents, teachers, and television are serious enough by themselves to cause tragedy or crime. What I want to bring out is the multiplicity of influences fostering excessive competitiveness, including the impact they are having on the less conscientious or less stable individuals, that are thus contributing to the progressive weakening of our society. For example, criminologists believe that a factor in our ever rising crime rates is that those youths who have no ideals because they've been neglected throughout childhood, seeing the fine things in advertisements and the high living in soap operas, say, "Why shouldn't I enjoy these things too?"

Among adults, the drive to maximize profits at all costs has led to insider trading crimes on Wall Street and to a baby food company selling sugar water as apple juice. Some athletes improve their performances with forbidden drugs. Some politicians take bribes to be able to win elections. Some bankers have wrecked their banks by making harebrained loans for high profits. Some leaders of nations have sacrificed the health and welfare of children and their mothers to win favor and election funds from industry.

I believe that the most vital force to counteract this trend is for parents (and also teachers) to raise children not to compete and get ahead, but to serve, to be kind, to be cooperative, to be affectionate. The most effective influence is for parents to treat each other and their children with consideration, respect and love, for young children are molding themselves all day long in the image of their parents.

In addition parents can encourage children to serve in ways that are appropriate to their age. Even two-year-olds can be allowed to set the table—and they want to do it because it's grown-up. Children of different ages should have regular duties in housework and yard work, not imposed in a killjoy manner but as ways to contribute to family welfare, preferably side by side with the parents. Adolescents should have regular jobs outside the home as helpers in children's institutions or as tutors of younger children having difficulties with lessons, or as sitters. Their experiences—successful and unsuccessful—should then be discussed in class with a mature teacher.

The spirit in which the parents assign jobs is crucial, not as unpleasant obligations but as opportunities to help other human beings—the parents always setting the example.

I do believe that if parents can see how competitively they work and live, and how they pass it on to their children, they can learn gradually to ease up, to get more enjoyment out of life, and to improve the neighborhood and the country at the same time. But it can only be done gradually and with effort at the start.

How Can You Judge Your Child's Teacher?

I'd say that the most important criterion by far is whether your child likes the teacher.

But, you may say, might a child like best a person who is not an effective teacher but who seeks popularity by being pleasant and making lessons too easy? That's a logical sounding fear, but it is not correct at all according to my experiences. In fact, children are quite critical of an undemanding teacher. I've heard them say, "Miss Jenkins is nice but she doesn't teach you anything."

Children learn best by identifying with an adult who likes them, and whom they like and admire. In the many parts of the world in which there are no schools at all, children learn hunting or fishing or agriculture or weaving or baby care or cooking by identifying enthusiastically with the parent of the same sex, whom they admire and love and want to grow up to be like. At the other end of the educational scale, we can see in a medical teaching hospital that the students and doctors in training are learning to be physicians by eagerly patterning themselves after the older staff doctors whom they admire—and who respect them. No students of any age want to pattern themselves after a teacher who doesn't like them.

When children like a teacher it means that the teacher loves them and tries to understand their individual problems. This is a major factor in successful teaching.

It's a mistake in general to think of the subjects children study in school as being difficult to learn and as therefore requiring unusual technical skill on the part of teachers, and hard work on the part of pupils. Subject matter at each grade level is relatively easy for a majority of pupils to learn without great effort, provided they don't get scared or blocked at certain points. They get blocked because they are scared of the teacher or scared that they don't and can't understand. So the friendliness and the patience of the teacher, in understanding where the learning block occurs and in helping them over it, are crucial elements in any teacher's capability.

Another reason why some children can't learn, of course, is because their learning capabilities are not up to the material presented in class because their intelligence is below average. A more frequent reason for a learning problem is seen in children who have difficulty learning in specific areas such as reading, spelling, arithmetic or writing. Often, the teacher's expectations are not realistic for these children, because they need special accommodations in the classroom to maximize their learning potential. For other children, problems with attention to learning tasks or unrecognized behavior problems may limit their learning.

I was in a small informal class of six students at the

age of eight years where the teacher, untrained, pushed me in a hurry to learn long division. It seemed so over-whelmingly complicated at that age that I wept every day. The fault there was that few children of that age are capable of long division.

"Learning capabilities" doesn't mean just intelli-gence. Ten percent of children in the early years of ele-mentary school who have good intelligence still are slow in being able to remember the shape and position of let-ters—they confuse "d" and "b" or they confuse "god" and "dog." This makes them, first of all, slow to learn to read but, even more damaging, is their loss of self-confidence and a feeling of panic that they won't ever be able to learn to read. Other children are slow in catching on to certain mathematical concepts. Such learning disabilities can be suspected by a well-trained teacher, diagnosed by tests, and treated by special methods.

To get back to judging teachers: a second sign of a good teacher, whether at the nursery school level or the high school level, is whether she or he spends most of the time talking at the whole class or spotting the indi-vidual who is stuck and helping that student to get unstuck.

One kind of poor teacher threatens students that she will give them low grades or not promote them. This is more likely to paralyze students who are falling behind than to stimulate them. The teacher's job is to make the work understandable enough, interesting enough, and challenging enough, so that the pupils can't help but get involved. This means designing projects, learning exercises, creative programs, and field trips that will make the subject matter seem real and exciting. It means giving serious students who are extra bright assignments that are extra challenging and giving slow students less difficult assignments so that they won't become discouraged but will get a sense of achievement every day. Of course, classes have to be small to make this possible. A teacher who uses physical punishment or sends a student to the principal for punishment has failed and has given up in my estimation.

A good teacher encourages initiative, responsibility and creativity. These qualities are essential to all students if they are to be ready to take on jobs in adulthood that are better than humdrum or bottom-of-the-ladder. These qualities can't be taught by books or by the preaching of the teacher—or by the parent. Children develop them by being given opportunities every day to carry them out in practice. The wise teacher gives her pupils daily opportunities to take the initiative, to make their own plans for some of their work, to try to solve certain problems by themselves—even if they make mistakes. She encourages them to be creative and original in their writing, in their art work, and in their dramatics. And after letting pupils plan some of their projects, she lets them carry these out with minimal supervision. You can only teach a child to take responsibility if you give responsibility.

How will you know whether a teacher is helping individuals, and is encouraging initiative, creativity, and responsibility? You may get hints and clues from what your child tells you about school. But best of all is to visit the classroom—not for a half hour but for at least half a day.

What if your child complains of a frightening teacher or one who can't seem to make the work understandable? It is particularly the sensitive, overly conscientious pupils, at the start of first or second grade, who are most apt to be overawed or scared by a teacher. They show this not only in their complaints about the teacher but, for some children, not being able to eat breakfast, complaining of belly aches only on school mornings, or vomiting on the way to school. This fear of not being able to satisfy the teacher at six or seven years is an aspect of the shift from being totally a child of the parents in the first five or six years of life, to beginning to be a person of the outside world where one has to cooperate, take responsibility and be increasingly independent.

I think it's helpful to listen sympathetically when a child complains of a teacher, but not to jump to the conclusion that the teacher is mean or incompetent. You can say, "I can see how that would upset you, to have the teacher scold you, in front of the class." Next you can offer to visit the classroom, to see what it's like. Just going there may tip the teacher off that there is some problem and make her more considerate of the child's feelings.

Next you could make an appointment for a conference, not to complain but to ask how the child is doing. Then you can refer to the problem, without putting it in terms of blaming the teacher: "He worries whether he can't do well enough" or "When he can't understand something right away, he gets panicky and gives up."

The overawed child usually gets a thickened skin in a few weeks and learns that the teacher's severity is not as dangerous as it seemed. If this does not happen and the child remains tense and unhappy, the parents can approach the principal for help. In this case it is just as important that the parents not put the blame mainly on the teacher, which usually forces the principal to defend the teacher. They can put it instead on the child's sensitivity or immaturity in development. A principal can read between the lines and may suggest some classroom accommodations for learning, a conference with the teacher or a formal evaluation by the school counselor or educational psychologist.

This discussion brings us two other issues. Parents with high standards and ambition for their children sometimes try to persuade a school to put their child in a higher grade or class than the school people feel is wise. This often proves a mistake because the child placed too high may be unable to keep up and then feels disgraced by being demoted.

Parents of an unusually bright child sometimes assume that he is bound to be bored in a class of average children. This isn't necessarily true at all. If the class is not large and the teacher is well-trained and imaginative, she should be able to enrich the child's assignments, for example with extra reading in the classroom, in the school library, or in the town library. This is the same principle used in the traditional one-room school, where there would be four or more grades in the same room and the teacher would assign different work to each child.

Lessons, Lessons

What about ballet and tap lessons, piano and violin lessons, drawing lessons, art appreciation and photography at the museum, opera appreciation? Are they valuable for children? Should children or their parents take the initiative in suggesting lessons?

I think it's valuable when children have one or two of these skills or at least an appreciation of such arts. A musical skill eventually gives deep pleasure to the performer and to others. It enriches the soul. It develops a sense of achievement. The same benefits come from skill in some form of dancing. In addition dancing is thought to develop poise and physical grace which I value.

To develop an appreciation for painting, drawing, sculpture, or photography will open doors of pleasure and inspiration wherever a person goes in life. The pleasure and inspiration will be intensified if the individual becomes an active artist, whether amateurish or skillful.

Some children in early and middle childhood take to music lessons so eagerly or have such inspiring teachers that they continue to practice conscientiously, without prodding by the parents. I've seen this most often in families in which there are skilled musicians who serve as role models and create a family attitude that considers it unthinkable to give up lessons or stop practicing once started.

But the biggest problem with music lessons for young children, it strikes me, is practice. I've seen the difficulty in friends' children and in my own, and heard about it often in patients. Children have no conception of how many months and years of dull practice it takes to be able to play at a level that gives pleasure. When parents, to test the depth of their children's interest, point out these difficulties, children brush the warnings aside and swear that they'll practice long and eagerly. Promises come easily in childhood.

Should the parent be the one to suggest lessons? I realize it will work in some cases, especially in lessons that don't require practicing. But considering how many children lose their enthusiasm after a while, especially for music lessons, my own prejudice is in favor of leaving the initiative to the child. Even that won't guarantee persistence; but children are more likely to stick to their practicing if the project was originally their idea rather than a parent's wish. I said this was "my own prejudice" because many parents choose to give their children the opportunity to try lessons in one of the arts. Each parent should decide what they are comfortable with.

The same philosophy of no parental pressure applies, in my mind if, after a few weeks or months, a young child says he doesn't want to practice or take lessons anymore. If the parents are very positive and tactful they may be able to persuade a child to continue. But I have a preference for stopping the lessons—for the benefit of the parents as well as child—if it becomes clear, over a period of months, that the child has lost all enthusiasm and is balking, despite the parents' and teachers' best efforts.

My opinion is that in any case it's preferable for the parents to avoid the job of reminding or pushing the child to practice. There are already too many other subtle sources of tension between children and parents, in most families. Let the pressure, if any is needed, come from the teacher.

I don't want my own pessimism about practicing to influence parents beyond a mild degree. I'm only reminding them of the problem in case they are skeptical of the child's dedication. But some young children do go on practicing and taking lessons, and eventually become capable musicians, through some combination of their own enthusiasm and of the teacher's and parents' encouragement or pressure. Who knows ahead of time which ones it will be? If you do decide to persevere despite only partial cooperation from your child, you can call it off later if you become convinced that you are losing rather than gaining ground.

I've been talking about individual music lessons and individual practice for young children at home. Now I want to shift the scene to the Suzuki method in which young children are taught and practice in a group as well as individually. Practicing in company takes a lot of the curse off it. The Suzuki method is also less of a chore for young children because they don't have to learn to read music in the beginning. It assumes that children will learn tunes the way they learn to speak, by imitation. Reading music can come later.

The situation in regard to music lessons is apt to shift in the high school years. If a school has a band and a system of instruction for musical instruments, many young people become interested in participating, through some combination of enjoyment of music, school spirit, and wanting to be in the social scene.

The intense interest in popular music that occurs in the adolescent years inspires some youths to resume music lessons that they dropped in earlier childhood, or to start lessons for the first time in instruments played in rock bands. Or they teach themselves. It may not be the kind of music that parents would have preferred, but it certainly inspires young people and satisfies their longings. Those who are adept may form their own bands. Some youths acquire an interest in classical music as they mature, as appreciators or as performers.

As for dancing lessons—ballet, tap, modern—many girls and some boys become interested and enthusiastic without any stimulation from their parents. If as a parent you are eager to have a daughter take lessons you would merely have to take her to watch a class once, if she is susceptible. If she isn't, I wouldn't urge her. I don't believe in children being pushed into activities because a parent thinks it's a good idea. Let the child take the initiative.

As for a child's possible interest in some aspect of art, you would probably have seen it already in the child's spontaneous drawings or paintings or clay sculpture. You can also take a child to art exhibitions about subjects likely to interest him, especially exhibitions of the work of children. Many children develop an interest in art when they watch an actual class of children at work. But let him decide whether he wants lessons.

I don't believe in tying up children's whole week in classes and activities. They should have free time for unorganized visiting with friends, for reading books not required by the school, for neighborhood games, and for hobbies. They should even have time for dreaming.

Index

abuse, child or spousal, 29,
44, 52–53, 248
academic work, pushing
preschoolers with, 25–26,
203–04, 248, 251–52
acceptance of others, 40
Action for Children's
Television, 55
adenoids, removal of, 112
adolescents, 140
communication with,
220–21, 222–23
drugs and, *see* drugs
friendships of, 215
parties, 236–37
peer pressure, 157–59,
216–25
pregnancies, 30, 44, 169,
170, 217
rules for, 183, 220, 221–22
sex education and, 168–69
sexuality, *see* sexuality
smoking by, *see* smoking
suicide among, 31, 218
youth culture, creation of,
161
Advertising Council, 56
affection, 38
after-school activities, 148–49
lessons, 149–50, 264–68
aggressive child, 216
bullies, 231–34
alcohol, 157, 158, 183, 217,
223–24
allowance, chores and, 33
American Broadcasting
Company (ABC), 56
anger, 189, 228
expressing parental, 188
anxieties, 43–44, 46
cartoons causing, 126–27
of grandparents, 113
of overprotective parents,
137
separation, *see* separation
anxiety
symptoms of, 191
apologizing for lying, 194, 195

appreciativeness, parental, 5, 33
apprehensiveness, 48–51
  parental, 70–71
argumentativeness, 17
arts, exposure to the, 264, 268
athletics, 253–54, 256
attention span, 126, 194

Baby and Child Care (Spock), xiii, xvii, 36, 153
"baby proofing," 137
babysitters, *see* sitters
beauty, 20, 24
bedtime, 174–75, 182
Bible, 41
birth control, 69, 170
birthdays, 8, 15, 128
birth order, 72–78
boarding school, sending stepchild to, 103
bossyness, 76
  of grandparent, 113–14
Boyd, Hilary, 105
breast feeding, 32
breathing of baby, noisy, 113
bullies, 231–34
  complaints about your child, 234

Cable News Network (CNN), 56
camp, summer, 119, 252–53
Canada, 85
career choices, 12
cartoons, 48, 151
  scary, 126–27
  violence in, 58, 151

causes for children, 42–46
Chanukah, 8, 15, 125
charity, 8–9, 84
cheerfulness, parental, 18–19
childbearing, age at, 31, 66–72
child care, *see* day care; sitters
chores, 257
  allowance and, 33
  spirit of enthusiasm and, 9–10, 11, 257
Christmas, 8–9, 15, 126
  gifts at, 125, 128–29
civil disobedience, 38, 46
close-knit communities, 21
clothing, 219
  getting dressed by oneself, 9
  grandmother's worries about warmth of, 111–12
  peer pressure and, 157, 218
coaches, 253
Columbia Broadcasting System (CBS), 56–57
comic books, violence in, 58
communication:
  with adolescents, 220–21, 222–23
  infant, 67–68
  sex education and, 64
community service, 8, 34
comparing one child with another, 77, 228–29
competitiveness, 250–58
  counteracting, 257
  overemphasis on, 25–27
  parental pressure and, 251–52, 253–54, 257–58

school grades and, 34–35, 252

second children and, 75

in sports, 253–54, 256

compliments, parental, 84, 230

concentration, 198

see also attention span

conforming to peer group, 157–59

consistency, parental, 34, 63

in discipline, 184–85

contemporary culture, 130–73

adolescent behavior, 157–64

aging and, 130–34

calling parents by first names, 152–57

decision-making skills and, 134–41

guilt about working outside the home, 141–46

sex education, *see* sex education

contraception, 69, 170

"cooking," 10–11

cooperation, 20, 32, 67, 142, 184

play and, 4, 6, 17, 201, 202, 204, 213–14

with stepparent, 99

counseling, 81, 157

for guilt about working outside the home, 145

for parent–grandparent conflicts, 115

for repetitive lying, 195–96

for self-critical child, 231

for stepchildren, 104–05

for unpopular child, 217

creativity, 15–16, 17, 135, 261

crime, 62, 256

theft or vandalism by neighborhood children, 236

criticism, 78, 107

of grandchild by grandparent, 117–18

by grandparent of parenting methods, 108–09, 112–18

of stepchild, 102, 104

cruelty, 7

crushes, 40, 42, 163

crying, 67–68

culture, changes in, *see* contemporary culture

curfews, 183

cursing, 172

dance lessons, 264, 267

Dante, 86

dating, 85, 86

by single parents, 95–96, 170–71

day care, 22–23, 44, 71, 214, 230

children's helpfulness and, 6–7

subsidies for, 61–62

"day nurseries," 22

decision-making, learning skills of, 134–41

demander-complainer, dealing with, 142–46

dependability of parents, 156

depression, 231
    separation anxiety exhi-
        bited as, 122
desensitization, 49, 53, 54, 58
Dewey, John, 241
diet:
    grandparents' beliefs
        about, 110, 112
    infant feeding, 32, 112
    see also meals
disagreeableness, parental, 5
discipline, 63, 174–96
    consistency in, 184–86
    father's role in, 186–90
    hesitancy in parents, 63,
        174–83
    for lying, 190–96
    rules, *see* rules
    setting limits, 17, 18
discrimination, 44
divorce, 23–24, 30, 171
    rates of, 81, 98
    youthful marriage and,
        81–82
    see also single parents
Dr. Spock's The First Two Years
    (Spock), xiv–xv
Down's Syndrome, 70
drugs, 44, 157, 158, 217, 219,
    223–24, 256
duties, *see* responsibility

eagerness, 11
education, 239–68
    academic work, pushing
        preschoolers with,
        25–26, 203–04, 248,
        251–52

competitiveness and,
    25–26, 34–35, 250–58
human relations as part of,
    242
incidental learning,
    245–50
"learning by doing,"
    241–42
lessons in music and the
    arts, 149–50, 264–68
medical school, 249–50,
    258
memorization and, 239,
    240–41, 249
in nonindustrial societies,
    239–40
sex education, *see* sex edu-
    cation
teachers, *see* teachers
see also schools
Einstein, Albert, 61
elderly, cultural changes and,
    130–34
enthusiasm, parental, 9–10
Europe, 85
expectations of behavior, 71,
    184, 192–93
extended families, 21, 178

fairness, parental, 156
faithfulness, parental, 2
families, 60–129
    changing, 60–66
    early or late childbearing,
        31, 66–72
    eating dinner together, 60
    extended, 21, 178
    favoritism, 77, 78–81, 205

first child, *see* first child

grandparents, *see* grandparents

help in minor crises, 33

holidays and, *see* holidays

importance of, 27–28, 60

making a difference, 65–66

nontraditional, 62

nuclear, 62

preparing children for a good marriage, *see* preparing children for a good marriage

science replacing spirituality, 64–65

second child, *see* second child

sex education and, 63–64, 164–73

single parents, *see* single parents

stepparents, *see* stepparenting

vacationing without children, *see* vacations

work and, *see* work

fathers as disciplinarians, 186–90

favoritism, parental, 77, 78–81, 205

fearfulness, 48–51

Federal Communications Commission (FCC), 56

firmness, parental, 18, 34, 63

first child, 229–30

    sensitivity of, 206

    sibling rivalry and, 205–06, 208

    sociability of, 211, 212–13, 230

first names, calling parents or adults by, 152–57

food, *see* diet

football, high-school, 253–54

forgiveness, 41

Freud, Sigmund, 165–66, 177

friendliness, *see* sociability

generosity, 1–9, 20, 38, 46, 129, 215

    love and, 1–2, 4–5

    readiness for, 3–8, 201–02

    special occasions and, 8–9

    spirituality and, 40, 42

    tolerance and, 7

getting ahead, 65, 255

gifts, 8, 84

    holidays and, 125, 128–29

    homemade, 129

    overindulgent parents and, 13–19

    thank-you letters for, 129

giving, *see* generosity

God, 21, 28, 39–40, 41

Gorer, Geoffrey, 28

grades, school, 243, 252

    competitiveness and, 34–35, 252

    of first child, 206

    second children and, 75

grandparents, 28, 105–18

    aging process, 130–34

    changes in pediatric practice and, 112

grandparents *(cont.)*
    conflicts with parents,
        108–10, 115–18
    grandmother, interfering,
        111–18
    holidays and, 127
    importance of, 105–11
    interfering, 108–18
    irritable, 106
    living with the family, 109
    needing emotional and
        physical support, 133
    security value of, 106
    in single-parent families,
        110
    as source of comfort, 108
    spoiling of grandchildren,
        107–08
Greece, 83
greediness, 8, 17, 84
    gifts and, 128–29
guilt, parental, 16–17, 136
    day care and, 22
    lack of love, 16, 80
    psychological revolution
        and, 178
    working outside the home
        and, 141–46
guns, 28–29

handicaps, feelings about,
    226–27
helpfulness, 5, 6, 32, 46
    opportunities for, 33
hesitancy of parents to disci-
    pline children, 63,
    174–83
hobbies, 143

holidays:
    gift-giving at, 125, 128–29
    grandparents and, 127
    manners at family gather-
        ings, 127
    relaxed, 125–29
    see also specific holidays
homework:
    creative, 135, 150–51
    repetitive, 135, 150
    sitters and, 147
honesty, 20, 42, 80–81
    lying, *see* lying
hospitalization, 51
    separation anxiety and,
        121
hostility, 76
household help, 6–7, 10–12,
    84
"house," playing, 6, 7, 9, 89,
    139, 166, 201, 202–03,
    247
How to Win as a Stepfamily
    (Visher and Visher), 105
humiliation, 35, 251

idealism, 20, 46, 64–65
identifying with parents, 38,
    144, 159, 211, 240, 258
    boys, 89–90, 189, 246
    generosity and, 3, 4
    girls, 90–91, 246–47
    political activism and,
        44–45
    responsibilities and, 9, 12
identity, searching for adult,
    157–58, 159
idols, teenage, 160–62, 163

imaginary parents, 89
imagination:
  imaginary playmates, 190,
    191, 192–93
  of preschoolers, 190–93
impatience, parental, 78–81
impressions, 34
incidental learning, 245–50
  versus school learning,
    249–50
indecision in child-rearing,
  parental, 174–83
independence, 2, 3, 104, 136,
  223
individualism, 255
individual sensitivity, *see* temperament
industriousness, 17
infant feeding, 32, 112
initiative, 17, 261
  fostering, 137–41, 151
  natural development of,
    136–37
  schools fostering, 135
insecurity, 62
insensitivity, 17, 53
interfering grandparents,
  108–18
intolerance, 7
Iran, 83
irritability, 106, 181, 207
Israel, 83

jealousy, 74
  sibling rivalry, 205–10
  of stepchildren, 99
Johnson, Lyndon, 32
joy of giving, 8–9

kindness, 20, 32, 65, 129
Kinsey Report, 165

"latchkey" children, 58, 141
leadership, parental, 153, 155
learning, *see* education;
  schools
"learning capabilities," 260
learning disabilities, 193
lessons, 149–50, 264–68
letter-writing, 38, 46
  thank-you notes, 129
library research, 135, 150, 242
limits, setting, 17, 18
lobbying, 38, 46
local and world problems,
  42–46, 84
love, 20, 32, 36, 39, 65, 129
  adolescent, 82, 163
  parental, *see* parental love
loyalty, 65
lying, 189–96
  apologizing for, 194, 195
  by preschoolers, 190–93
  by school-age children,
    193–96
  see also honesty

making a difference, 65–66
manners, 139, 209
  at holiday gatherings, 127
marriage:
  age at, 31, 68–69
  preparation for, *see* prepar-
    ing children for a good
    marriage
  remarriage, 24, 97–98, 171
materialism, 27–28, 65

meals:
    coming in for, 175, 182–83
    eating dinner together as a
        family, 60
    responsibility for food
        preparation, 10–11
    see also diet
meanness, 76
Media Action Research
    Center (MARC), 55
Medicaid, 131
medical school training,
    249–50, 258
Medicare, 131, 132
memorization, 239, 240–41,
    249
menstruation, 167
mental retardation, 113
moral authority of parents,
    237–38
morals, 40
Motion Picture Association of
    America, 56
movies:
    sexuality in, 30, 36, 171–72,
        219
    violence in, 29, 36, 47–69
murder, 29, 44
    television and, 49, 53
music lessons, 149–50,
    264–68

National Broadcasting
    Company (NBC), 57
National Coalition on
    Television Violence, 55
negative associations,
    parental, 79

neighborhood children,
    231–38
    bullies, 231–34
    moral authority in control-
        ling, 237–38
    parties and, 236–37
    robbery or vandalism by,
        236
    at your home, setting limits
        for, 234–36
news media:
    tragedies in, 42–44, 47–59
    see also television
nightmares, 191
"nontraditional" households,
    62
nuclear family, 62
nursery school, 71, 214,
    230

only child, 151
    imaginary playmates, 192
optimism, cause for, 31–32
orphanages, 88–89
overindulgent parents, 8,
    13–19, 135–36
    creativity and, 15–16
    expectations of children
        and, 83
    lack of appreciation and,
        15
    lack of hesitation and,
        18–19
    limits and, 17, 18
    older parents, 70
    parental guilt and, 16–17,
        136
    reasons for, 16

sacrifice and, 14
selfishness and, 17–18
sharing expenses and, 15
in the U.S., 14
vacillation and, 18, 19
overscheduling, 146–52
after-school programs,
148–49
children's views about, 147,
149–52
decision-making skills and,
134–35
letting children select activities, 148, 152

pacifiers, 112
pals, parents acting like, 155,
156, 188
panic, 49
"parallel" play, 4, 202, 208
"parental hesitancy," 63,
174–83
parental love, 38, 156, 184,
228, 231, 257
favoritism, 77, 78–81, 205
generosity and, 1–2, 4–5
guilt over lack of, 16, 80
second child and, 76
Parenting, xiv
parties, 236–37
passivity, 134, 135
pediatric practice, changes in,
112
peer groups:
adolescent peer pressure,
157–59, 216–25
identification with, 3, 7, 39,
45

imitating, 139
perfection, striving for, 27
permissiveness, 153
persecuted child, 216
personality, 210–11
birth order and, 72–78
of interfering grand-
mother, 113–14
physical development, progression of, 113
see also social development
Piaget, Jean, 200
play:
academics stressed over, in
preschoolers, 25–26,
203–04, 248, 251–52
adult concept of, 187–89
cooperative, 4, 6, 17, 201,
202, 204, 213–14
"house," playing, 6, 7, 9,
89, 139, 166, 201,
202–03, 247
individual pace of mastering skills of, 200
"parallel," 4, 202, 208
parental participation in
child's, 200–01
sharing, readiness for, 4, 6,
201–02
of six-to-twelve-month
infant, 199
as work of early childhood,
197–204
"playing" with children, 144
police, 51, 236
politeness, 32, 33, 34
political activism, 32, 36–38,
44–46, 84–85, 255

popularity:
    helping the unpopular
        child, 210–16
    valuing, 211–12
    see also peer groups
possessiveness, 4, 5, 6, 201–02
praise, 138
prayer, 42
preaching, parental, 32–33
pregnancies:
    teenage, 30, 44, 169, 170,
        217
    Victorian attitudes, 164
preparing children for a good
        marriage, 81–88, 225
    discussions with parents
        and, 85
    divorce ratios, 81
    entitlement and, 83
    expectation and, 83–84
    later marriage and, 82
    living together and, 82–83
    marriage to the wrong
        person, 86–87
    parental role models and,
        87–88
    political activism and,
        84–85
    sexuality and, 85–86, 225
    youthful marriage, 81–82
preschool, 71, 214, 230
presents, *see* gifts
Presley, Elvis, 161–62
pressures, 25–27
    adolescent peer pressure,
        157–59, 216–25
    competitiveness, *see* com-
        petitiveness

preteens, *see* adolescents
pride, 21
programming for children,
        55–57
promiscuity, 168
psychological counseling, *see*
        counseling
psychological revolution:
    Freud, *see* Freud, Sigmund
    parental confusion caused
        by, 176–78, 180
psychosomatic diseases, 250
P.T.A. meetings, 135, 244
puberty, 162, 167
punishment, 5, 35–36, 63,
        261
punk look, 157

"quality time," 142

Rambo, 54
rape, 29, 53
rashes, baby, 113
reading to your child, 194, 248
rebelliousness, 40, 41, 45, 159,
        160, 217, 218
Redbook, xiv
religious beliefs, 20, 28,
        39–42, 218
    see also spirituality
remarriage, 24, 97–98, 171
    see also stepparenting
resentment, 77–78, 184
    of stepchildren, 99
respect, 17, 35, 38, 58, 154,
        210
    calling parents or adult by
        first names and, 154, 156

responsibility, 9–13, 257, 261
  food preparation, 10–11
  ideal of service and, 33,
    257
  parental role models and,
    12
  schools fostering, 135
  spirit of enthusiasm and,
    9–10, 257
  suggestions at each age, 13
robbery by neighborhood
  children, 236
role models, 10, 12, 42, 173
  see also identifying with par-
    ents; preparing children
    for a good marriage
rudeness, 75, 142, 156, 184
  to stepparent, 99, 100, 102
rules, 184–86, 219
  for adolescents, 183, 220,
    221–22

sacrifice, 14, 61
salvation, 41
"sandwich generation," 133
Scandinavia, 17
scheduling, *see* overscheduling
schools:
  after-school activities,
    148–49
  age to start learning, 252
  boarding, sending
    stepchild to, 103
  choosing between, 244
  class size, 147–48, 242, 261
  dropout rate, 243
  grade and class placement,
    proper, 263–64

  homework, *see* homework
  lying about schoolwork,
    190, 193, 194
  motivations for learning,
    243–44
  parental involvement with,
    244, 262
  philosophy of, 135, 147–48
  poor grades, 193–94
  sex education in, 168,
    242–43
  teachers, *see* teachers
  see also education
science, spirituality replaced
  by, 21, 64–65
science projects, 135
scolding, parental, 32–33, 34,
  80, 84
second child, 72–78, 212–13
  sibling rivalry, 75, 205–06
security:
  grandparents, provided by,
    106
self-centeredness, 17
self-criticism, 235–31
self-doubts, 226–31
self-esteem, parental role in
  child's, 226–31
selfishness, 17–18, 129
self-respect, 17
sensitivity, 48–51, 84
separation anxiety, 120–24,
  191
service, ideal of, 32–39,
  64–66, 257
  community service, 34
  duties at home and, 33
  in foreign countries, 83

service, ideal of *(cont.)*
  political activism, 36–38
  punishment and, 35–36
  school grades and, 34–35
  violence and, 36
sex education, 29–30
  age-appropriate, 167–69
  parental role, 63–64,
    164–73
  in school, 168, 242–43
  sexual awareness of
    children, 165–66,
    167
  single parents and, 97,
    170–71
  in Victorian era, 164–65
  see also sexuality
sexism, 69
sexuality, 216–17
  casual attitude toward sex-
    ual activity, 169–70
  early stages of sexual devel-
    opment, 157, 158,
    162–64
  Freudian theories, *see*
    Freud, Sigmund
  in the media, 30, 36,
    171–72, 219
  peer pressure and, 224–25
  preparation for marriage
    and, 85–86, 225
  promiscuity, 168
  of single parents, 170–71
  spiritualism and, 29–30,
    172, 242–43
  see also sex education
shaming, 230
sharing, *see* generosity

shyness, 212, 216
sibling rivalry, 205–10
  first child and, 205–06,
    208
  handling quarrels, 209, 210
  parents' contribution to,
    207–08
  second child and, 205–06
siblings, 5
  caring for, 12
  comparisons between, 77,
    228–29
  hypercritical attitude
    toward, 68
  imitating, 9
  loving one child less,
    78–81, 205
  lying to, 194
  second child, 72–78
  single children wishing for,
    151
sin, 41
single parents, 88–98
  children in two-parent fam-
    ilies and, 88–91
  contact with live-apart par-
    ent, 92–93
  dating and, 95–96, 170–71
  grandparents' importance,
    110
  joint custody, 72
  mothers being good
    fathers, 96–97
  no contact with live-apart
    parent, 93–94
  references to absent par-
    ent, 92–94
  remarriage, 97–98

sexual relationships,
170–71
substitute parents and,
91–92, 94–95
sitters, 147
separation anxiety and,
122, 124
slang, teenage, 222
sleep, 151
bedtime, 174–75, 182
nightmares, 191
smoking, 157, 158, 218,
223–24
sociability:
of first child, 211–13, 230
promoting, 212–16,
233–34
of second child, 75, 213
social development, 197–238
adolescent peer pressure,
157–59, 216–25
holiday gatherings and,
127–28
negative comparisons, children's, 226–31
neighborhood children
and, see neighborhood
children
play as work of early childhood, 113–14
sibling rivalry, 205–10
the unpopular child,
210–16
see also physical development, progression of
Social Security, 131, 132
soul, 65
spanking, 35

"spirit," parental, 9–10
spirituality, 30–31, 38, 39–42
loss of, 19–22, 129
materialism and, 27
science replacing, 2, 64–65
sexuality and, 29–30, 172,
242–43
Spock, Mary Morgan, xvi–xvii,
99–105
spoiling of grandchildren,
107–08
see also overindulgent
parents
spontaneous helpfulness, 4
sports, 253–54, 256
stepparenting, 24, 98–105
being compared to natural
parent, 102–03
being overly critical of
stepchild, 102, 104
books on, 105
jealousy and resentment,
stepchild's, 99
personal experiences with,
99–105
rudeness of stepchild, 99,
100, 102
time before relationship
improves, 103–04
Step-parents' Survival Guide, The
(Boyd), 105
stresses, 19–22
subsidies, government or
industry, 61–62
substitute parents, 91–92,
94–95
suicide, 231
teen, 31, 218

summer camp, 119, 252–53
Sunday school, 41, 42
Surgeon General of the Public Health Service, 54
Suzuki method, 266–67

teachers, 147–48, 243, 244, 252
    expectations of, 258–59
    fear of stern, 244, 262–63
    how to judge, 258–64
teenagers, *see* adolescents
television:
    amount of time spent watching, 134
    forbidding children to watch, 49–52, 57–59
    scourges on, 42–44
    sexuality on, 30, 36
    supervising children's viewing, 54
    violence on, 29, 36, 47–59
temperament, 48–49, 72, 159, 194, 210–11, 229, 233
Thanksgiving, 127
thank-you letters, 129
theft by neighborhood children, 236
Three Stooges, The, 52
timidity, 48–49, 212, 216
toilet training, 112
tolerance, 7, 38, 40, 42
tonsils, removal of, 112
tragedies, 42–43, 47–59
trust of your child, demonstrating, 195, 221

unconventional behavior, 46
understanding, 40
ungratefulness, 17
United States, 14
    competitiveness in, 251
    lack of child-rearing traditions in, 179
    political activism in, 17–18

vacations:
    separation anxiety and, 120–24
    without the children, 118–24
vacillation, 18, 19, 57
values, 1–59
    cause for optimism, 31–32
    causes for children, 42–46
    competition and, *see* competitiveness
    duties and responsibilities, *see* responsibility
    giving and sharing, *see* generosity
    materialism and, 27–28
    overindulgence and, *see* greediness; overindulgent parents
    parents working outside of the home, 22–23
    religion and, *see* religious beliefs
    service, *see* service, ideal of
    sexuality, *see* sexuality
    spirituality and, *see* spirituality
    stresses and, 19–22

unsatisfactory work and, 24–25

violence and, *see* violence

vandalism by neighborhood children, 236

venereal disease, 169

victims, identifying with, 43, 48, 51

Victorian attitudes toward sex, 164–65

Vietnam era, 32

violence, 36, 47–59, 209–10
cartoon, 58, 151
child abuse and, 52–53
desensitization, 49, 53, 54, 58
fearfulness and, 48–49
forbidding children to watch, 49–52, 57–59
parental action against, 54–59
playing at, 52
reassurance about, 50–51
talking about, 50

tolerance of, 28–29

Visher, Emily and John, 105

volunteerism, 8, 46

voting, 37, 45–46, 65–66

Watson, John, 177

winning, importance of, 27

withdrawn child, 216

women's liberation movement, 68

work, 255
adult distinction between play and, 187, 188–89
incidental learning about, 247–48
overemphasis on, 60–61, 255–56
parental guilt about, 141–46
urban versus rural, 83
without satisfaction, 24–25
women and, 68–72

world and local problems, 42–46, 84

LOOK FOR THE COMPANION VOLUME:

DR. SPOCK'S
THE FIRST TWO YEARS

The Emotional and Physical Needs of
Children from Birth to Age Two

Contents

**1. Communicating with Your Baby:
Reading Your Baby's Cues**

Crying: An Early Form of Communication with
Parents • Baby Colic • Periodic Irritable Baby •
Fretful Baby • Cries of Hunger • Hypertonic Baby •
Crying Associated with Diaper Rash and Teething •
Responding to Your Baby's Cry: A Few Specific
Suggestions • Is the Baby Sick? • Sucking •
Reaching Out • Kicking Legs • Grunting •
High-pitched Squealing • The Parent's Response •
Happy to Crying • Enjoy Your Baby

2. Parents' Biggest Newborn Concerns

Umbilical Stump • Floppy Head • SIDS • Exposure
to Germs • Breast-feeding • Swelling of Babies'

Heads • Breathing Patterns • Soft Spot • Playing
Too Vigorously • Spitting Up • Jaundice

3. Choosing a Doctor for Your Baby

4. The Arrival of the New Baby

Feeding and Behavior • Breast-feeding • Formula
feeding • Preparing for the New Baby • Preparing
Sibling for the New Baby • Preparing the Parents
for the New Baby • Arranging Help for Mom • If I
Have a Baby Boy Should He Be Circumcised?

5. How Much Regularity to Infant Feeding?

When a Mother Thinks About
Going Back to Work

6. Beginning Solids

Which Solids, in What Order?

7. Poor Eaters

8. Common Physical Problems

Teething • Sneezing, Coughing, and
Dripping . . . the Common Cold • Ear Infections

9. Stranger Anxiety

10. Transitional Object

Thumb-sucking

11. Sleep Problems

Newborns • Six to Sixteen Months: Demanding and Walking • Naps: Six Months to Two Years • Co-sleeping: Children Sleeping in the Parents' Bed • Bedtime Rituals • Bottle in the Bed: Age Six to Twenty-four Months • Separation Anxiety: Six Months to Six Years

12. Toilet Training

13. Discipline and Temper Tantrums: An Opportunity for Parent–Child Communication and Learning

Anger and Temper Tantrum

Physical Punishment

Humiliation, Shame, and Guilt

14. Can You Spoil a Child?